Reflections on Diabetes

"I had him look into the lives of men
as though into a mirror, and from others
to take an example for himself."
—Terence

"A moment's insight is sometimes worth
a life's experience."
—Oliver Wendell Holmes, Sr.

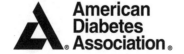

**American
Diabetes
Association**

Publisher	Susan H. Lau
Editorial Director	Peter Banks
Editor and designer	Sherrye Landrum
Cover art	Jack Pardue
Cover design	Renee S. Boudreau
Illustrations	Tacy Judd
Desktop publishing	Sherrye Landrum
Production Director	Carolyn Segree

Printed in the United States of America

American Diabetes Association, Inc.

1660 Duke Street
Alexandria, VA 22314

Library of Congress Cataloging-in-Publication Data

Reflections on diabetes.
     p. cm.
"A Diabetes Forecast book."
ISBN 0-945448-65-1 (paper)
1. Diabetes--Patients--United States--Biography. I. American
Diabetes Association

RC660.4.R44   1996
362.1'96462--dc20   96-6157
                                          CIP

Table of Contents

Travel, Sports, and Adventures

Taking Charge

Friends and Lovers

Preface

This is a book of short stories—stories by and about people who live with diabetes every day—which first appeared in *Diabetes Forecast* magazine. Health-care professionals usually think about diabetes in terms of clinical concepts, such as blood glucose levels, insulin dosage, and calorie intake. The situation is very different for those who live with diabetes on a daily basis. Although clinical concepts are important to people with diabetes (and to those who care about them), living with diabetes is much more than concepts and numbers. Diabetes is woven into the emotional, intellectual, spiritual, and physical fabric of their lives. For those touched by it, diabetes becomes a part of their life story.

Although these authors have never met each other, they have some things in common. First, they have all been touched by diabetes in ways that have proven challenging and sometimes painful. More than that, they share the bond of people who have learned from the experience of living with diabetes. They are stronger and wiser, not just from having diabetes, but from allowing the experience to teach them important lessons about themselves and about life. Finally, they are all people who are willing to allow others to share in their lives and their learning.

We, the readers, owe them a debt of gratitude for being open enough to share their struggles, pain, successes, and, most of all, their hard-won insights and commitment to meeting the challenge of living well with diabetes.

Robert M. Anderson, EdD

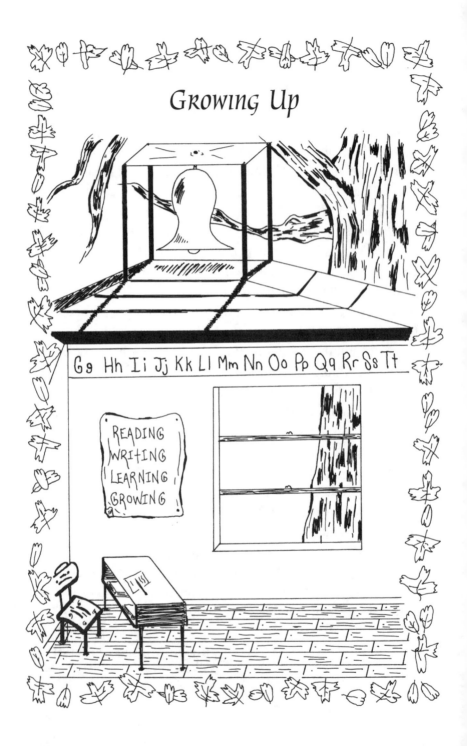

Growing Up

Who's the Counselor Here?

by Sarah M. Mart

I survived my freshman year at the University of
Montana, but by the end of the first session of summer
school, my candle had nearly burned out. Socially and
academically, my first year looked like a success: a high
grade point average, lots of new friends, and extracurricular activities I really enjoyed. In my quest for success,
however, there remained one factor in my life I ignored:
my diabetes.

Perhaps "ignored" is too strong a word. I always took
my injections within one or two hours of the time they
should have been taken and I never hid my diabetes from
anyone. But in a college student's hectic life, who has time
to test four times a day? Who wants to eat exactly what she
should eat, exactly when she should eat it? When a bunch
of friends want pizza at 3 o'clock in the morning, who
refuses?

Who indeed? But as these rationalizations became
more and more common, I found myself forced to ask
some tougher questions. Why was my insulin dosage
increasing, and why had my cholesterol levels doubled in
one year? Why was I losing weight? Why didn't I feel
well?

These questions pounded away at me as I filled out my
application to be a counselor at my alma mater of summer
camps, Camp Diamont in Montana. Having spent seven of

the happiest weeks of my life as a camper there, I planned to return as long as I could. But this year, uncertainties and doubts plagued me. Who was I to tell these kids what to do when I had had such a feeble grip on my own control? What kind of role model could I possibly be?

That last question caused me to begin to change my habits. And although I realized some truths for myself, and hopefully taught the campers a little, they taught me quite a bit.

I learned that I do not fail at my diabetes when my blood glucose reads higher than desired. I simply cannot let one reading ruin my attitude! At school I skipped testing when I knew it would read high, because I did not want to see the large number. I listened to myself as I repeated to my cabin of 12-year-old girls, "A reading is not good or bad. It is only a number." After preaching that for a week, I finally began to practice it!

I learned that nothing cures the blues faster than an 8-year-old boy, who disdains all members of the opposite sex, tackling me out of nowhere to give me an enormous hug because, "well . . . you're okay for a girl." And that an adolescent girl asking to borrow my clothes or makeup is offering the ultimate form of acceptance.

I learned that no matter how many peanut butter and jelly sandwiches I took to the cabin at bedtime, the number would be at least one less than the number of girls reading low at 2 a.m. And that no matter how long someone has diabetes, every once in a while it feels nice to have someone else give the shot.

I also learned that no matter what my G.P.A. says, or how many honors classes I take, I pass a real test of success when I can stand up in front of a hundred people and make up aerobics to "Wild Women Do"— when I as a rule usually do not. I discovered that to be called "way cool" by a munchkin-sized bunch of people is just as important as a test grade, and in many ways, is more fulfilling; and most important, that I am not alone with this disease.

Thanks to camp, I know more than 100 people I can write or call to help me survive whatever crisis I find myself facing. Proof of this occurred one day when, monitoring everyone else's tests and shots, I forgot my own. Three voices chirped, "Did you do your shot? What was your test? Are you low?" They reminded me that I must take care of myself and keep my priorities straight.

My week at camp rearranged those priorities and taught me a lesson more important than any other I learned during my first year at college: This disease is part of me in the same way my brown eyes or love of music are. I must not only accept it, but do my best to incorporate it into my life. Camp continues to be the best way I know to help me do that. As one of my fellow counselors told me this year, "I skipped camp one year. It was the worst mistake I ever made." I understand why he feels that way.

I now know that my sophomore year at college will be successful. I simply needed to redefine success in my own terms.

Whaτ Neeδles Me Abouτ Havιng Dιaberes

by Sally A. Hedman

"Do you have to give yourself shots?"

"Yeah."

"Where?"

"Usually in my arm, leg, or stomach."

"Your *stomach*? Doesn't it hurt?"

"Well, sometimes it does, when I hit a sore muscle or a blood vessel."

"I could never give myself a shot in the stomach. I'd pass out."

Since I was diagnosed with diabetes more than six years ago, I have engaged in this conversation countless times. You know, diabetes gives me some really challenging things to do like eat a special diet, constantly monitor my blood sugars, and lead a life that is rather controlled. But this conversation sums up the typical reaction I get whenever I tell people that I have diabetes.

When people say that they could never give themselves shots, I think they aren't listening to themselves.

Although some seem pretty impressed that this has become as routine for me as brushing my teeth, others, by the looks on their faces, have a mental image of a 4-inch needle as thick as a pencil that I have to stick in my body. They don't want to know any more.

Besides, everyone does things to stay healthy. This is

one of the things I do to stay healthy. Don't people realize that not injecting myself would be really irresponsible? If they actually had diabetes, would they really rather suffer uncontrolled diabetes with dry-as-cotton mouth, endless trips to the bathroom, plummeting weight, fatigue—and those are just the fun parts—or would they administer those injections just like I do?

Most people mean well, I know, but hearing the same thing over and over again can get old. For once, I would love to be asked if there are other ways I control the disease, like diet or exercise. Why does everyone focus on needles and shots? Isn't anyone impressed that I can control a disease like diabetes? And still lead a somewhat normal life for a 23-year-old woman?

Most people don't know I have diabetes until they offer me a piece of candy, a cookie, or a piece of gum. My question: "Is it sugar-free?"

"Dieting?" they ask.

"Nope," I say, "I have diabetes." Then we do the shot routine. And after that, most people go on to declare that they simply Would Not Survive if they were denied their daily candy bar, and how can I stand not eating candy?

This is the other thing people seem to know about diabetes. I explain that I can eat candy, but only when my blood sugar is low, not just when I have a craving. (Many times—especially if the person has an obvious weight problem—I would love to answer, "I'm glad I have to watch my diet and exercise, you might want to try it yourself.")

I know it's hard for anyone who doesn't have diabetes to know how it feels, but it might help if everyone knew just a little more about it.

I have been controlling this disease for a few years with some success. But when I'm at home, my parents seem to want to make my disease theirs. When dinner is being prepared, someone will say, "Don't forget to take your shot, Sally." Right. Glad you reminded me, but it's not something that is likely to slip my mind. (Sharing this disease is a tricky process.)

Thanks to my parents, I have a library of books about diabetes and a lifetime membership to the American Diabetes Association. I have all the information I need at my fingertips, and I want to share it.

I know that most people—even my parents—are curious, and things like shots are unfamiliar to them, so they ask questions. The problem is no one ever comes up with new ones.

I have yet to encounter an original response to the news that I have diabetes. Maybe I should start the ball rolling and say something positive to the next person I meet who has diabetes. If what goes around comes around, someday I may finally hear someone say, "You have diabetes? Is that why you're in such great shape?"

Editor's note: The new dietary guidelines recommend that you have a meal plan developed to fit your lifestyle. Sugar is a carbohydrate that can be included as part of your meal plan.

DISCOVERING INDEPENDENCE

by Laura Partin

It was August, and I was eager to begin my first year of
college. I felt like a typical freshman: excited to try out
new freedoms and responsibilities, but fearful of failure
and rejection.

These self-conscious fears added to my growing anxiety
about being on my own. My parents had always been there
to help with decisions about my daily insulin adjustments.
Now, responsibility for my health was on my shoulders
alone, or so it felt.

My first major decision was who to tell about my
diabetes. In high school, my peers treated me no
differently after my diagnosis than before. But I wondered
whether my new dorm mates and classmates would be as
accommodating.

I didn't wait long to find out. Within the first five
minutes of moving in, I told my roommate and resident
assistant (RA) about my diabetes. I briefly explained what
it is, what I have to do to live a healthy life, and how to
treat low blood sugar reactions. They were receptive: My
roommate's father was a doctor, and she found my condition
"interesting." My RA's reaction was a low-key "okay."
That helped ease my fears of rejection.

Within a few months, I was confident enough to give a
talk about my diabetes in speech class. I'm glad I did. As a
result of an eight-minute speech, I opened a wonderful

dialogue with two classmates. One also had diabetes, and another had a diabetic parent and grandparent. For the other students, I had placed a face on an otherwise abstract disease.

Throughout much of the semester, my diabetes management progressed just as smoothly. It wasn't until late November that my new independence was really put to the test.

A few friends invited me to go on our semiregular, five-mile walk to stay in shape. I was a little hesitant because I had not eaten all of my dinner, but I thought if I tested before and after I exercised, I would be fine. The blood test read 72, so I drank some fruit juice and ate a small sandwich before I left.

The first mile was relaxing and fun, but after the second mile, I suddenly wasn't feeling very well. I hurried back to my room to test again. As I suspected: 58.

I shakily poured myself a half glass of fruit juice and sat down to do my math homework. Or at least I tried. I couldn't get my mind to work fast enough and the numbers began to blur. It had been 15 minutes since I drank the juice.

I checked again: 48.

"Ugh," I thought, "I better drink some more juice and eat a bagel." I ate the food, realizing I was not even hungry, but my blood sugar called. I waited another 15 minutes and decided to test again, just to be safe: 69. "Good," I said to myself, and finished my homework.

But as I put away my math book, I didn't feel so well again. I tried to stand up, but my legs had forgotten how. I very carefully crawled over to my food stash. After I drank some more juice and ate something, I decided to call for help. I made it to the phone, but I couldn't get my fingers to dial. Nor could I remember anyone's number.

I pulled myself toward the door, but I passed out about halfway there. As I felt my body go limp, my brain yelled, "Move!" I lay there awhile drifting in and out of consciousness. Eventually, I mustered up enough strength to make it to the door and force my body halfway into the hall.

My RA discovered me. She began to ask me the questions I had taught her. "Are you having a sugar low?" "Do you need food or a sugar shot?" I shook my head "yes" or "no" in response to her questions, at least the ones I could comprehend. She ran to her room, quickly returned with fruit juice and chocolate, and helped me drink the juice.

I felt myself coming back around, and I began to cry. I had tried so hard all semester to be completely independent and carefree. Now I was completely embarrassed. And frightened.

I tested a few more times that night, but the ordeal was over. As I got ready for bed, I realized I would always need people like my RA to be there for me, like guardian angels.

But what about my independence? I remembered the burden of feeling all alone, and I began to understand.

True independence is not freedom from other people. Rather, it's allowing others to watch out for me, while I do the same for them.

A Glance in the Mirror

by Amy J. Neil

I never knew how he felt.

He masked his pain at my diagnosis of type I diabetes with a calm smile. "We'll tackle this together," he told me. "I can help you handle it."

And so he asks, with each weekly telephone call, "Been feeling OK?"

"Fine!" I tell him—even if I'm not. After all, I don't want to worry him.

"Have you been eating all right?" he asks.

"Yes," I reply. I do not want to be questioned. I do not want to be bothered. I must handle this myself.

He is always careful not to ask me too much or to pressure me about my disease. Still, I can't help feeling a loss of privacy and independence when he asks specifically about my blood sugars or inquires about my diet. I know that it is up to me to adopt the behaviors that will help me control this disease, despite helpful advice from him and others. The consequences of poor control—lethargy, malaise, the threat of complications—are my true motivations for self-care.

When we discuss my diabetes, he listens patiently. Yet our efforts to "protect" one another from the worries and fears we both feel resemble a well-strategized chess match: each side carefully maneuvering to avoid direct confrontation—the confrontation of fear and other emotional and physical burdens of chronic illness.

I thought I knew how he felt. The "concerned parent," I reasoned. "Be patient. Realize it's difficult for him to watch, relatively helplessly, while his daughter struggles with this illness." I tried to understand. I shared the positive aspects with him: good reports from the doctors, new discoveries of personal strength and resilience I never knew I possessed. But I continually tried to shield him from the negatives. Another move in the chess match.

When I visited last Christmas, I knew immediately.

"Dad has diabetes, doesn't he?" I asked Mom.

"Yes. He was just diagnosed with type II diabetes. But don't tell him that you know. He doesn't want to worry you children."

I was angry. Why wouldn't he discuss it? It would be easier for the family to handle the moods, his sudden fatigue, and his uncharacteristically somber disposition, if we could talk about diabetes openly. After all, we also are affected by this disease. I was hurt, worried. "We can help him handle it," I thought. I didn't want to see him combat this alone. I knew the family could be an important source of support.

But I remained silent. When I was diagnosed, I had battled these same feelings of frustration and denial, and I had resisted his help. I knew I had to let him handle his diabetes, as he had let me handle my own. Still, I watch with concern when he doesn't appear to be feeling well.

"Feeling OK?" I ask.

"Fine!" he replies, even if he isn't.

I suddenly understood, more clearly than ever, the worries and frustration he must have felt as I struggled to control my illness. I know that no matter what I say or do, only he can control his diabetes.

We all are responsible for handling our disease, primarily for ourselves but also for those we love. Our loved ones are a vital source of help and support, but they can't direct our self-care efforts. They can only watch and hope that we care for ourselves properly.

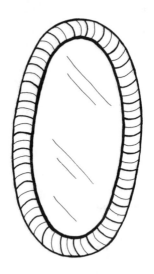

"You know," my father confided one day, "I hate it when I don't feel well. I'm just not used to it. I've been healthy all my life."

"I know," I said. I knew we both understood.

And so, in our own way, my father and I have begun to communicate our feelings. We now share the special bond of fighting the same adversary. He knows how I have felt these last 10 years coping with type I diabetes, and I know how he felt watching me. My father's diagnosis was a glance in the mirror for me.

Now, I know how he feels.

THE WALL

by Lurette Kerr

When I was diagnosed with type I diabetes at age 18, I became suddenly, keenly aware of having joined the ranks of the "handicapped," the "limited," the "flawed." Driving home from the doctor's office, my mother advised me to keep "our secret," for my condition would cost me friends, suitors, and jobs. At our Thanksgiving family gathering, my aunts and uncles spoke in hushed tones of my "condition" and thanked God for the remaining "whole" offspring in the clan.

Insulin dependent, "impaired," I no longer belonged to the Whole World. There was a wall dividing the Perfect People and the Compromised People. My Medic Alert necklace flashed my disability: DIABETIC. I could not eat, play, work, or even sleep without consideration of my limitation. My body didn't work properly. I was defective.

The wall between me and the Perfect People seemed so obvious, so solid, so sturdy. I was struggling along with others who were "abnormal" and dependent to succeed in the world of the healthy and independent.

Of course, I was always happy to see a "fellow flawed" succeeding in the Whole World. One morning I was half-watching a news program while putting on make-up. I paused, mascara wand in hand, and gave my full attention to a legless man who was competing in a marathon. The TV camera focused on the man's powerful arms directing his wheelchair across the finish line. "Good job," I thought, grinning. "You gave the Perfect People a run for their money!"

Mascara wand still suspended, I watched the newscaster interview one of the winning runners. The tall athlete turned his head aside, sneezed, and said, "My allergies nearly got me—the pollen is out early this year!" His face was puffy; he struggled for breath.

The newscaster shifted his microphone to another finisher's face. "I ran this one for my Pop," beamed the athlete. "He couldn't be here today cuz he's in the hospital recovering from a cancer operation."

The newscaster held the microphone up to a third winner. "How's it feel to win?" he asked.

The runner grinned, "Good, man, good! And I wanna say something to Dickie—that's my kid brother. I wanna say 'Dickie, there's more than one way to win!' You see," he confided, "Dickie isn't used to his big brother's winning. I'm dyslexic, can't read. But I can run!"

The camera panned the sunlit crowd. There was a very obese woman standing next to a man with hearing aids. A hyperactive little boy twisted himself around a restraining rail. A woman with bottle-glass spectacles peered into the sun. For a moment, I thought I recognized an old classmate—a girl who had been diagnosed as manic depressive in college. The man beside her looked like my coworker— a chain smoker who couldn't quit even after his wife died of emphysema.

The camera drew back and reduced the newscaster and the crowd to a generic microcosm of humanity. Then, during the commercial break, a parade of laxatives, antacids, and pain killers danced across the screen.

"Good grief, where are the Perfect People?" I thought. Who do I know who isn't struggling against migraine headaches, arthritis, addictions, or personality afflictions? Was the single mother with shattered self-esteem or the victim of eating disorders any more whole than I?

Suddenly I couldn't find any Perfect People to put on the other side of the wall. I couldn't find any Uncompromised People. After years of thinking diabetes separated me from a privileged class of people without problems, I felt myself merging into a vast array of variously limited, variously challenged human beings.

The wall was gone. I realized that wholeness is not a gift divinely bestowed upon a lucky few; it is, rather, something achieved by those who choose to face life's challenges head on.

We earn wholeness when we see life's obstacles not as walls, but as hurdles. With each hurdle that we jump, we come that much closer to fully realizing our true potential.

Six Years

by Katie McGovern

S weet is not the adjective that usually comes to mind
when referring to insulin-dependent diabetes, but I
would describe my six years of living with diabetes as at
least bittersweet. I've had to face an unexpected illness,
decide whether or not to let others know about it, and find
a way to deal with the ignorance of others about diabetes
in general.

My days of insulin shots and blood tests began when I
was eleven. Surrounded by my friends and teachers at a
sixth grade campout in a remote Virginia forest, I displayed
the classic symptoms of untreated diabetes. At dinner, I traded my spaghetti, bread, and dessert for cartons of milk and
juice, drinking a total of seven. That night I staggered from
the cabin to the outhouse so many times that I lost count.
My face was bluish-gray, and my frail body shook from the
cold despite the sleeping bags my friends piled on me.

I left camp early, and within 24 hours I was in the
hospital. In five days, I learned how to do my daily insulin
injections and blood tests, but I was not ready to accept
responsibility for my health or talk openly about my
diabetes.

When I returned to school, everyone wanted to know
what had happened to me. Rumors about my illness flew,
aided by the school secretary who, thinking she was pro-
tecting my privacy, told my class that I had something that

"would never go away." At first I had a really hard time saying "I have diabetes," and would only tell people who directly asked. I often let my best friend speak for me.

It wasn't until seventh grade that I learned the price for keeping my diabetes a "state secret." One day at lunch a guy I had a crush on stood up in the cafeteria and loudly accused me of giving myself shots. Immediately friends I hadn't confided in leapt to my defense, shouting back that it wasn't true. I realized then that people will take their cue from me. If I act as though diabetes is something to be ashamed of, it's only reasonable that others will see it that way too.

I was finally able to begin accepting my disease when I went to diabetes camp. Although I disliked many things about the extremely regimented camp, I learned there that I was not a diabetic, but a person with diabetes. My disease does not define me.

The moment that made all the extra food measuring and intense blood sugar monitoring at camp worth it came during a doctor's lecture. A counselor who did not have diabetes asked a question and referred to kids who didn't have diabetes as normal. Another counselor who had diabetes jumped to her feet and chewed out the first counselor for implying that people with diabetes are abnormal. I realized then that I had been seeing myself as less competent than people without diabetes. I had been allowing the disease to take away my opportunities. I learned that having diabetes didn't mean I couldn't travel to another country by myself, backpack in a remote area, or go on other adventures.

I admired the strength of that outspoken camp counselor, and, in ninth grade, my own resolve to educate people about diabetes was put to the test. My misguided biology teacher told what he considered a humorous story about his high school band instructor who had diabetes. When the instructor had an insulin reaction, he would go wild, his conductor's baton flying faster and faster. My teacher also expressed concern that his neighbor's daughter would become diabetic because she drank a lot of cola. At that point, I was forced to decide between revealing my diabetes to a class full of strangers or allowing my teacher's insensitivity and misinformation about the causes of diabetes to go unanswered. I raised my hand.

I've changed a lot. Now, when someone notices my Medic Alert bracelet or when it's time to do a shot, I give a standard lesson in diabetes management to those around me. Once I show a willingness to explain my disease, people usually have many questions to ask.

People with diabetes sometimes talk about being grateful for their disease because of all they have learned from it. Although not a day goes by without my wishing that I didn't have diabetes, I know what they mean.

Having diabetes has helped me recognize that I am responsible for taking care of my own health. It's taught me to be assertive in the face of both curiosity and ignorance, and to define myself as a human being and not as a disease. I've also learned never to let the "limitations" of diabetes become self-fulfilling prophecies. In short, I'm ready to face whatever life has to offer.

Parenting

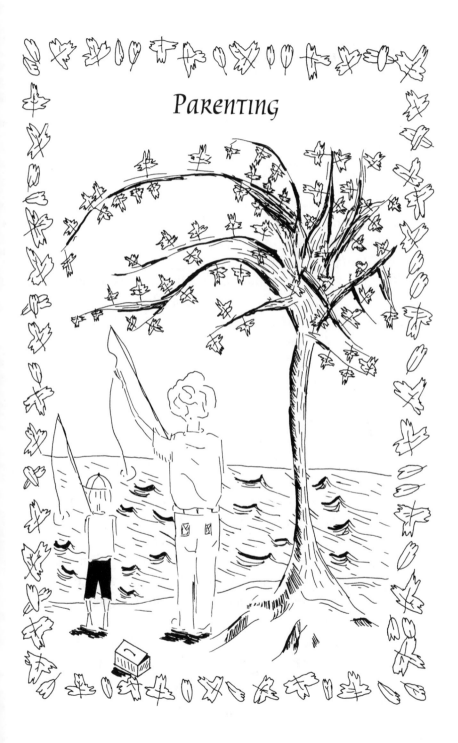

I Can Live With It

by Bonnie Jones Graham

Fourteen years ago, our first child, Seth, was born. My husband, Thomas, and I bought Dr. Spock's book and loaded up on pacifiers. Seth slept through the night on day 1. After 18 months, I tossed out the unused pacifiers and propped up a crooked table with Dr. Spock's book.

Had I been superstitious, the fact that our next child, Heidi, was born on Halloween might have been a sign. She didn't stop crying for three years. Food-induced allergies left our little spook miserable, itchy, and squalling.

I took out a loan for pacifiers and experienced the true meaning of sleep walking. After six months, I simultaneously discovered goat's milk, windup swings, and wax ear plugs.

Two and one-half years later Laura was born. She couldn't get enough air into her little lungs to do more than whimper, she was so badly affected by inhalant allergies.

We moved from soggy Seattle to Anchorage. Laura thrived in the cold Alaskan climate, and Heidi was weaned onto "real" milk. Thomas and I stopped subsidizing goat farmers and cleared six months without a hospital bill. We slept eight uninterrupted hours for the first time in years.

Then, three years ago, it happened: Our son, Seth, the healthy one, was in Anchorage's Providence Hospital. Diagnosis: diabetes.

"You can live with it, Bonnie," said my friend Sandy, whose daughter had developed type I diabetes when she was a toddler. The tears swelled in my eyes. Sandy was crying, too.

I discovered there was no cure, and I still have not told Seth that he will never fulfill his dream of being an Air Force pilot and astronaut.

I purged our kitchen of chocolate chips and potato chips and threw my old, chipped dishes at the wall. I ate chocolate-covered peanuts in my bedroom closet, and my belly ached as badly as my heart. I memorized Kubler-Ross's five stages of grief and did them all. Except one. Acceptance.

While my heart went through a wringer, Seth coped surprisingly well. He pricked his finger four times a day for blood sugar counts and drew his insulin into syringes and worried more about playing Nintendo than injecting himself twice a day.

Yet, Sandy's words continued to echo in my ears. "You can live with it, Bonnie." I couldn't see how.

Seth had his first diabetic emergency several months after he was diagnosed. He lost consciousness while eating a peanut butter and sugarless jelly sandwich and fell off a kitchen stool. I couldn't find the square boxes of juice and I had tossed out all the sugary stuff. My neighbor ran over with her kid's trick-or-treat loot. The cat ate the sandwich, and the candy brought Seth back to me. The next morning I went to the store and bought a sack of sugar. And more chocolate-covered peanuts.

On his birthday, we discovered that candles melt when set into hot pizza. Along with sputtering flames, he blew multicolored puddles of wax all over our dinner. We sang Happy Birthday anyway and ate waxy pepperoni pizza and created wild and crazy ideas for future pseudo-birthday cakes. We laughed ourselves sick until we realized we were laughing again, and I learned people really can laugh and cry at the same time.

We taught the girls how to call 911, and we discussed insulin pumps and pancreas transplants as casually as our plans for dinner and slope conditions at Alyeska.

Seth and I went bowling. I ate chocolate-covered peanuts, he drank diet cola, and we held an intense competition for the Graham gutter-ball championship. I won. I don't know how it had happened, but we were living with it.

A few weeks ago, Seth invited his two best friends, Willie and Issac, over. I popped my head in to tell him dinner was ready, the signal to take an injection. Our bowling scoresheet and a crumpled chocolate-covered peanut bag were stuck to his bulletin board alongside the space shuttle patch he had received from an astronaut.

The girls were building a Lego castle on the floor. Willie was sitting on the bed defeating Nintendo villains. Issac cracked jokes about Seth's future earning power as a human pincushion. Sandwiched between them, Seth pulled out his needles and insulin. While helping Willie negotiate a brick wall on the TV screen and telling Issac to zip his lips, Seth rolled up his sleeve, gave himself a shot, and flicked a Lego piece at his sister's head. With an artfulness born of much practice, he snapped the needle off the syringe and winged the entire thing into the trash can across the room.

No one noticed. Except me.

Editor's note: The new dietary guidelines recommend that you have a meal plan developed to fit your lifestyle. Sugar is a carbohydrate that can be included as part of your meal plan.

Checking Pockets

by Cynthia Cotten

Have you ever noticed that, no matter how carefully you go through pockets on laundry day, you always miss one tissue? The result at the end of the cycle is bits of damp shredded paper all over your clean clothes. You shake each item out as you put it into the dryer, hoping the lint catcher will take care of the bits that don't drop off. But somewhere there's a mess, whether inside the washer or on the floor of the laundry room. So you clean it up, resolving to be more thorough about checking pockets next time.

You check pockets in other areas of your life, too. You go through them from time to time, trying to empty them of anything that might create a mess. If you're careful, you can do a pretty good job. Most of the time.

If you have kids, you find yourself wanting to be more vigilant about checking pockets, both literally and figuratively. If you don't check the real pockets, Lord only knows what's going to go through the washer. How about Chapsticks, library cards, the occasional coin or two, and maybe a crayon, just to keep things interesting. As for those other kinds of pockets, you do the best you can. You get the kids vaccinated, you warn them not to talk to strangers, you teach them about the evils of presweetened cereal and too many Saturday morning cartoons. You hold your breath the first time you watch them climb a big tree, or jump off the diving board into the deep end. You pray a lot. And you try not to think about how messy it could get if you've missed a crucial pocket.

In November 1991, my twelve-year-old daughter was unexpectedly diagnosed as having type I diabetes. It was then that I realized there are some pockets that I can't possibly check because I don't even know they are there. This pocket's contents created a mess that turned my life upside down, and while I was trying to clean up, the mess was made worse by overpowering feelings of anger, fear, sadness, and frustration. There was no guilty party I could point a finger at and say, "Why didn't you check more carefully?" Oh sure, in theory I've always known I couldn't protect my kids from everything. But I didn't know how difficult and painful an experience it would be to discover the truth behind that theory.

In the emergency room that November night, so many doctors asked me the same questions over and over that eventually I could answer before I was asked. Yes, she had been drinking a lot, eating more, and complaining of feeling tired. But there had been a logical explanation for each of those symptoms: it had been hot, and we all drank a lot; she was growing fast; it was the start of a new school year. Diabetes had never occurred to me. There was no record of anyone ever having had it in either my family or my husband's. But even so, in the back of my mind, a little voice kept whispering, "You missed one...."

In those first months I saw my daughter's diabetes as an oversized, unwieldy garment, loaded with pockets. Some had to be checked daily. Her blood sugar levels had to be tested three or four times between breakfast and bedtime. Did she have snack stuff in her purse? Did I need to buy test strips, or lancets, or any other of her myriad necessary supplies? At school, we had to be sure her teachers knew about diabetes, about what to do in case she had a hypoglycemic episode and, in the worst-case scenario, how to use glucagon.

I'd always been a label reader; now my favorite recipes had to be carefully scrutinized. When we traveled, I checked to be sure there was a loaf of bread, a jar of peanut butter, and some fruit juice in the car, "just in case." Even if we were just out for the day, we had to keep her eating schedule in mind and check the time periodically. The number of pockets in this garment seemed endless, and for a long time I lived in fear that the one I forgot to check would be the one with the tissue in it. I didn't want to contemplate the mess that it could create.

Now, though, after a year and a half, either the garment has shrunk from daily use or—more likely—I've grown. In any case, it doesn't seem quite as overwhelming as it did when it was new. And life goes on, as it always does. Like all parents, I survive the occasional missed pocket and the ensuing mess. I have to. Because, no matter how unpleasant or inconvenient it might be, no matter how we rail against it, mess is a part of life.

Fine, I can accept that. But I'm not going to leave those pockets alone. Just because I know messes will occur doesn't mean I enjoy them.

So I'll keep checking.

Nothing is as Sweet as Mom

by Clifford J. Heaphy, EdD

When I was diagnosed with diabetes in 1967, an endocrinologist told my mother that she must be overprotective if I were to survive. My mom heeded not a word. As soon as she arrived at my hospital room, she instructed the nurses not to coddle me too much. I think she suggested that I could do floors and windows, but I can't prove that now!

Mother campaigned to let me live normally. (Well, she thought I was special, but not because I had diabetes, but because I was me!) I simply had a health condition that needed to be dealt with in a positive manner.

She started her own educational program to inform people about diabetes. She fought the Boy Scouts, school coaches, and anyone else who wanted to ostracize me because I had diabetes. I could do anything that any other boy could do.

Mother's attempts to normalize my life did not always meet with success. One example was her sugarless fudge. This recipe was provided by a dietitian who was full of creative suggestions like "sour cream can take the place of whipped cream and fudge doesn't need sugar." Sugarless fudge wasn't a culinary delight, but it did make a great toy for my younger siblings, and later helped re-tar the roof!

When cyclamates were about to be removed from the market, Mom took her hidden household money and purchased 20 cases of my favorite diet cola. All the other kids drank real colas, so it was my one compensation. She stored the stockpile in the storeroom outside—a move we later regretted when an unusual cold wave hit—the cans froze and exploded.

She never criticized me or my attempts to be a normal child, even though she did interfere when I tried to convince my best friend's mother that marshmallows really were a Bread Exchange on my diet!

It was Mom who always managed to keep a sense of humor when there seemed little to laugh about. When I went through a series of flu hospitalizations with ketoacidosis in 1976, she stood many hours outside the intensive care unit (ICU). The drive from our house to the hospital was clocked at speeds that would impress the Unser brothers!

When yet another 24-hour episode of vomiting and diarrhea hit, I resisted going to the hospital again. Mom took me anyway, and the doctors in the emergency room, who were working to reverse my dehydration, announced I was again headed for the ICU. "ICU???" I quavered.

"I see you, too," Mom quipped, to calm my fears. The roomful of professionals stopped to look at this crazy lady who was joking with her child in critical condition. I wish I had been able to tell them that she was really saying, "Honey, you have been there before, and you'll beat it again. Your Dad and I will be there by your side."

When I developed retinopathy, she went with me to daily clinic visits and a series of laser treatments that were then painful, difficult, and frightening. (Now the whole procedure is much easier.) After one visit, I left the clinic with both eyes bandaged. Mom talked all the way out to the car, reassuring me that people were not staring at me and everything was OK.

My door lock was jammed and she had to go around to her side to let me in the car. But she didn't. Instead, I heard her voice trail off as she drove out of the parking space. I stood there, bandaged and wondering when she would realize I wasn't in the car. Then I heard the brakes. She put the car in reverse and backed up. I could hear the evening news: Blind child with diabetes run over by emotional mother in hospital parking lot—film at 11! She managed to reach me without running over my toes. We both laughed all the way home.

She let me go to face the world, but her door is always open if I need a haven to come to and regroup. She let me make my own mistakes and choose my own goals. Most of all, she has shown me how rich life can be when it is lived—every day—with humor and love.

You're Not Alone

by Kimberly Evanovich

I'd read story after story about parents and their diabetic children, but none came close to my experience. It seemed that in each story, the parents accepted their child's diagnosis of diabetes with strength and dignity, learned everything there was to learn, and passed all of this information along to their receptive and responsible diabetic child. I couldn't help thinking, "What's wrong with us?"

Shane was only five when he was diagnosed. I learned what I could and felt committed to helping my son live a healthy life, but I was in no way prepared for how he would react to his condition. Whenever it was time for his shot, he cried, screamed, and hid. He called me names and accused me of hating him. No matter what I packed for his lunch or cooked for dinner, he hated it. And testing his blood was a nightmare. He had to be bribed with special treats or toys to cooperate, and the readings were almost always too high or too low.

It wasn't long before I felt completely overwhelmed and alone. Whenever I took Shane to the pediatric diabetes center, the doctors scolded me for Shane's unstable blood-sugar values. They responded to my despair and confusion by referring the entire problem to a dietitian, who would ask Shane what he liked to eat. He'd reply cheerfully, "Salmon, french fries, and spaghetti!"

This really meant that Shane might eat one of these foods if they were provided to him within five minutes, before he changed his mind again. But the dietitian would reply almost sarcastically, "I don't suppose your mother should have any trouble getting you those things to eat." Then, handing me a chart listing food exchanges (of which I had literally dozens at home), she would say, "If you follow these guidelines, his blood sugar values should stabilize within a few weeks." I always left feeling discouraged, guilty, and hopeless.

Until I met Dr. Bloome.

A change of insurance carriers required me to select a new pediatrician. On the day of our first visit with Dr. Bloome, Shane came home from school with a blood sugar of 456. (He had traded lunches with another boy.) His injection sites were flabby and his index fingers were covered with what looked like hundreds of black dots. I was at wit's end.

Dr. Bloome immediately took charge. Instead of treating Shane like a poor victim of maternal irresponsibility, he got right down to Shane's level and asked him point blank, "What is going on here?"

Shane was definitely taken aback by Dr. Bloome's forceful personality, as was I, but Shane actually seemed to be paying attention. By the end of the visit Shane had agreed to cooperate at injection time and "think about" doing his own blood test. I had been given the assignment of reading some books I hadn't heard of before and looking into a diabetes camp. Before we left the office, Dr. Bloome looked me straight in the eyes and said, "By the end of six months I want you to be teaching me things."

When we returned the next week, Shane met a 12-year-old girl who told him about doing her own shots. She even showed him her markless fingers, which Shane thoughtfully compared to his own dot-to-dot versions. Dr. Bloome pointed out to Shane that this girl was once just as out of control as Shane, that many times she'd had blood sugars so high the meter wouldn't even read them. "Oh yes," the girl's mother added, "I couldn't get her to take her condition seriously for years. All of our other doctors blamed me."

I was amazed. This was the first time I had ever heard of someone else having the same problems as I did. The other mother gave me her phone number, "just in case I ever needed someone to talk to," and I just about burst into tears. For once, I didn't feel hopeless and alone.

A few months after meeting Dr. Bloome, Shane was doing his own blood tests, without complaint, three or four times a day, and he was helping me chart the results and adjust his dosage. Not long after that he started to do his own injections, and his eating habits improved dramatically. He also had a great experience at diabetes camp, where he made friends and gained a new level of self-confidence.

Dr. Bloome was not a miracle worker; he just showed us how to find our way out of the maze of confusion and self-doubt we had wandered into. For me, the biggest change came from realizing that I was not alone. I was not a "bad mother" because my son's diabetes was out of control. I had the confidence as a parent to insist that we gain control over this disease. And together, we did.

Laughing Through It

by Bev Jarmenko

A kid who's newly diagnosed with diabetes has a hard time, as my 12-year-old daughter, Debbie, can tell you. But it's not so easy on a mother, either.

When Debbie first learned to inject herself about a year ago, she practiced on pillowcases and had to do dastardly things to stuffed rabbits. At the hospital, I learned the injection routine too, but the first time I held a syringe, I got nervous giggles and then panicked. Somehow the insulin I was holding mysteriously disappeared from the syringe, probably shooting into the carpet. I worried I looked like an unfit mother. Debbie got good at injecting way before I did.

We began testing her blood at home. There was the first shock of discovering that when it's cold outside, no blood comes—she was relieved to learn that this does not mean she is "empty." One time she pricked a hole in her finger and it wouldn't bleed, but blood suddenly spurted from an earlier finger prick. Eventually, however, even this shedding of blood became routine.

Blood testing is no small skill. She could enter the Guinness Book for mistakes made. Surely putting a drop of blood onto a strip and waiting 60 seconds could not be too hard. But we dropped the strip onto a wet table. The timer battery fell out. The blood drop wasn't big enough. The blood drop didn't hit the center of the strip. Once, we took the meter with us on an outing and forgot the strips.

But through it all Debbie found humor in the situation. She'd set the timer secretly behind me and then leave the room so it would beep later and make me jump. She played with two timers, setting them to beat in unison, creating a little melody.

We learned a new way of life—the food plan. The good news is that now she gets to eat six times a day. The bad news is that each meal looks like doll food. In our family, where juice and cheese used to be the allowed pigouts, here we are suddenly measuring them by the gram.

The kitchen is now cluttered with wall and fridge notes—emergency procedures, juice equivalents, weights of common things, cookie equivalents, emergency phone numbers. The house has become diabetized just as years before it had been kid-proofed.

The diabetes cookbooks were a real enigma. Why is it they offer a rich treasure of things like Zucchini Saute and Meat-stuffed Eggplant? Who wrote that amusing little section on how to make whipped cream, chocolate sauce, and jelly, all without sugar? Why is it that diabetes happens to the very people who love sweets the most?

Food begins to take on more importance than ever before. It was a heartbreaker when the two precious chocolate chip cookies Debbie was allowed on the picnic fell into the lake. One school morning I noticed that Debbie had forgotten her cheese allotment, and I ran all the way after her, into the school, waving the cheese and calling to her. She was mortified.

There was even that time I made Debbie sink into the floor when I had the deli clerk measure the popcorn.

But forgive me—I am new to all this. I'm always talking about how diabetes is no trouble and we can adjust, and it's no big deal, but heaven help the poor kid when she comes home and I learn that she has had her dinner an hour and a half early, without even injecting her insulin.

I now have a list of how much spinach and creamed corn Debbie can eat, but she refuses to touch the vegetables. I eat them all, feigning delight at radish roses, zucchini, and alfalfa sprouts. But there is a heartening discovery here: Debbie may have diabetes, but she's still a kid.

She's passed her latest swim level. She's getting acclimated to the trampoline. She's learned to enjoy a bit of tea and coffee.

We've learned diabetes is not all bad. When she meets other kids with diabetes, there's a brilliant flash of Medic Alert bracelets, like precious jewels. There's the camaraderie of riding in a bike-a-thon fundraiser. There's the reassurance that because of her strict diet, she'll probably never get fat, never get zits. And she'll always be skilled at measuring things, and chances are that she'll always be punctual and organized.

I don't know what it is about diabetes. I hate that she has it. I wish if someone had to have it, it would have been me. Once, when registering her for a course, my eyes welled up with tears, out of the blue, when I had to fill out the section on her medical conditions. I realize that I am poorly equipped to handle this. But by some miracle, she is not.

Editor's note: The new dietary guidelines recommend that you have a meal plan developed to fit your lifestyle. Sugar is a carbohydrate that can be included as part of your meal plan.

Almonds and Raisins

by Evelyne Pytka

When I was a child, and the ups and downs of life
overwhelmed me, my mother used to try to comfort
me with an old Jewish saying: Life is a mixture of almonds
and raisins—the bitter and the sweet. It didn't mean much
to me at the time, but now that I am a mother of three and
have developed diabetes, I understand what she meant.

From the time of conception, through pregnancy and
childbirth, and then on to the struggles of childhood and
adolescence, parenting is truly a concoction of almonds
and raisins. Parents of children with chronic illnesses and
disabilities know the taste of almonds and raisins, particularly the almonds.

But what about parents who themselves suffer from
chronic illnesses such as diabetes, especially mothers, who
still tend to be the primary caregivers in our society? As
a mother with diabetes, I have tasted many almonds and
raisins while trying to balance my obligations as a care-
giver with my responsibilities for my own health.

Since I developed diabetes almost three years ago,
another of my mother's sayings has taken on a new meaning: A mother always saves that last piece of bread for her
children. I know that a mother is supposed to be selfless, but
a mother with diabetes must also be selfish. I have had to
learn, and so has my family, that there must always be a last
piece of bread for me. There are some things even a mother

can't share, like the juice boxes and granola bars I keep stashed in my purse, coat pockets, and glove box in the car. When I was diagnosed with type I diabetes, I was advised about exercise and hypoglycemia. I was told that housecleaning, walking, bicycling, and other forms of exercise made it necessary for me to either eat more food or take less insulin. No one ever mentioned boisterous play with my children, a trip to the playground, or even sleepless nights spent nursing a sick child. After I experienced hypoglycemia in situations that I never would have considered as "extra activities," any outing alone with my children began to assume terrifying proportions.

At the time of my diagnosis, my children were 1 1/2, 5, and 7 1/2, and required a good deal of my time. Like most children, they were eager to participate in many activities. But good diabetes management also takes time: time to test, evaluate, inject, and, of course, eat! (Have you ever noticed how many extracurricular activities coincide with meal times?) During that first year of insulin injections, my children had to taste a few almonds: They participated in no extra activities—that was the only way I could cope.

Since then, I have switched to multiple injections. I now have greater flexibility, and my children have extra activities again. Gradually, I am developing a new sense of normalcy. I have learned that living with diabetes can still include old passions such as cross-country skiing and playing and teaching the violin. Diabetes has also inspired me to see some old pastimes and chores in a new light. I love to cook, and my new knowledge about good nutrition and food choices is helping me to create a cookbook.

Still, my greatest challenge is balancing my responsibilities. I know that better blood glucose control will help reduce my chances of developing complications. But tight control robs me of spontaneity and it can prove dangerous when I have to deal with the sudden changes and altered plans that are part of life with children. My dilemma is that I would like to ensure that I will be around to enjoy grand-children, and yet I want to be a full participant in life now.

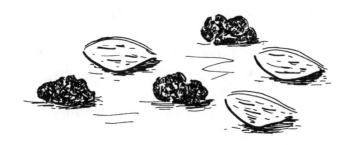

Although my life with diabetes does seem full of almonds, there are some raisins, too. Life tastes sweet indeed, when every Halloween my children set aside some of their sweets for "Mommy's Emergency Kit," or when my youngest daughter bakes an imaginary chocolate cake "with no sugar." My family has learned how to respond and help me when my blood sugars are low, and not to be offended by my behavior when my blood sugars are too high. Everyone now understands why I must carry a purse that resembles a well-stocked pantry.

As living proof of my mother's old bittersweet saying, the members of my family—who can't always come first—keep finding more raisins to offer me.

And do they ever taste sweet.

Giving Life, Living Life

by Lisa Barton

My husband and I have our second beautiful baby now, and we are so happy! I am also happy to report that I had a normal second pregnancy, and that our baby is as healthy as can be.

Well, it was almost a normal pregnancy. I was diagnosed with type I (insulin-dependent) diabetes between the births of my two children.

Because of the diabetes I had to take a few more precautions the second time around. And, of course, I did have some apprehensions about the safety of the baby I was carrying. But I have to admit they were not much different from those I had when I was carrying Emily. I think it is only natural to worry about the health of your unborn child—whether you have diabetes or not.

Some friends believed that by becoming pregnant I put myself and my baby in jeopardy. That is just not so. I am not saying that diabetes is a low-risk disease. But speaking from experience, I know that it's a disease that can be controlled with proper lifestyle, habits, and diet. I fervently hope that I will never decide to lead my life differently because I have diabetes.

I know that some people with diabetes are forced to make adjustments in their lives. I think they should do everything that can be done to ensure proper control of the disease, and then LIVE LIFE!

It is often difficult to change people's perceptions of what can and cannot be done. That's why I feel a responsibility as a woman with diabetes who has delivered a normal baby to let people know that, while diabetes is inconvenient, it need not alter your lifestyle in the all-important area of having a family.

Actually, in many ways my second pregnancy was easier than my first. I was terribly sick the first time, while the second time seemed to fly by! I felt well rested and had no bouts of nausea as I had had before. And, while I know that it is not uncommon for women to have different child-carrying experiences, I believe this proves my point. In the 1990s, there should not be any fear that pregnancy is radically different for the woman with diabetes as the one without it.

I did attend a pre-conception counseling clinic before the second pregnancy. Doctors there stressed one thing: Have a normal blood glucose reading for a time, along with a normal glycated hemoglobin test before becoming pregnant. (This is a test that reflects the average blood sugar for the past six to eight weeks.) Becoming pregnant when your diabetes is out of control complicates the pregnancy.

I have worked at maintaining good blood-glucose control ever since I was first diagnosed with diabetes. It only makes good sense to me, since high or low readings only serve to mix me up emotionally and make me physically tired. I have every incentive to maintain good control.

Once my good control was confirmed, attending the pre-conception clinic became only a routine check-in with my endocrinologist and obstetrician. And it was very convenient to see a gynecologist before becoming pregnant, because there were a lot of questions I wanted to ask.

Then mid-pregnancy I visited my endocrinologist and obstetrician every two to three weeks. The main reason was to ensure that as my body changed, my medications could also be changed.

Late in the pregnancy I had stress tests as often as twice a week, confirming that all was well in the womb. Of course, the frequency of these tests sometimes made them tiring, but it was worth it when Sarah Marie Barton was born on September 29, 1990, weighing in at 8 lbs. 10 oz.

For me, pregnancy seemed to confirm so much about what is good in life. Raising a family makes me feel I am doing something vital for myself and my husband as well as my community. I feel a direct contributor to life! And when I realize this, a contentment with my lot steals over me and I realize how lucky I truly am.

LEARNING DAYS

by Barclay Marcell

October 12, 1993 My hands shake involuntarily as I weave through the afternoon rush hour traffic. I glance furtively at my 5-year-old son, Jared, who sits in the front seat beside me pressing buttons on his Ninja Turtle hand-held game.

Just a few moments ago we had been sitting in the pediatrician's office, where Jared's blood sugar level registered over 800. I had the feeling that from that moment on I would divide our family's life into two discernible time frames—Before Diabetes and After Diabetes. The former period seemed a time of relative innocence.

November 10, 1993 "No blood check! No shot!" Jared buries his head deeper into the pillow, hiding his hands under his body so I can't reach a finger. "Jared, please let me do this." Reluctantly, his tussled head emerges and he produces an index finger. I can see the little marks along its tip—the result of the four daily pricks over the last month. I try to find an unused spot and then without delay press the trigger on the lancing device. Jared flinches. Thankfully, I got enough blood for an accurate reading.

I squeeze the fatty part on the back of his arm, trying to avoid a bruised area where I previously hit a capillary. Jared squirms and reaches over with his free arm. "Not yet!" he pleads. Undaunted, I poke the needle in as quickly as possible to minimize the pain. I depress slowly and then withdraw. Jared and I both breathe audibly. All of a sudden he's a different kid, running toward his box of Ninja Turtles as if nothing has taken place. I, on the other hand, feel drained.

December 15, 1993 Last night I had my recurring dream again. It usually takes the form of Jared stuffing his face with sugar-laden Twinkies and chocolate bars while I look on helplessly. This particular dream involved my mother, who was assuring me not to worry as she whisked Jared off to a bakery. As her station wagon pulled away, I looked at my watch, knowing that it was past time for Jared's insulin injection.

February 20, 1994 Jared's monitor reads 294, the highest reading he's had since his diagnosis. How could this be? I think back on the morning's food choices. Was it the "sugar-free" granola bar I'd given him for his 10 a.m. snack?

Jared seems to feel fine and eagerly awaits his lunch, but I'm depressed. When will I reach the point where my moods do not swing up and down according to Jared's blood sugar readings? If we go through a whole day with readings within our designated target range, I feel elated. If his levels go above or below this range, then I feel I have somehow failed.

March 19, 1994 Yesterday, I acted for a brief time as though Jared's diabetes did not exist. He had already eaten his morning snack and was playing with his friends while I made lunch. One child said she was hungry, so I brought out a bowl of chips for the kids to munch on while I finished up in the kitchen.

"*Pleeese*, can I have some?" Jared pleaded with me. "*Pleeese!*"

The other kids were devouring the chips and I thought, what harm can a few chips do? In essence, I was hoping that, maybe, just this once, Jared could be like the other children. But when I pricked his finger before lunch, the extra chips (and I believe he had more than a few hand-fuls) had caused his blood sugar to rise to 240. Our one mistake seemed to set the tone for the afternoon and evening as his remaining readings all registered on the high side. A lesson learned.

April 12, 1994 It's now been 6 months since Jared's diagnosis, and I'm beginning to find ways to deal with the frustration, anxiety, and guilt. I've read books that recom-mend each day be approached as a clean slate. You do the absolute best job that you can and try not to succumb to the self-blame which only makes it more difficult to get back on track. I also try to remind myself that things usual-ly do go well. And I cherish moments of insight, such as the time I saw Jared through the eyes of his best buddy, Michael.

Michael was at our house playing when we did a blood check. As Jared wiped the excess blood from his finger, he exclaimed, "Hey, that didn't even hurt!" Michael stared at him with obvious admiration. "You're the bravest guy I know," he said. But Jared seemed not to have heard and ran off to continue their karate game.

Tears welled up in my eyes. I turned to Michael and said, "He *is* brave, isn't he."

Complications

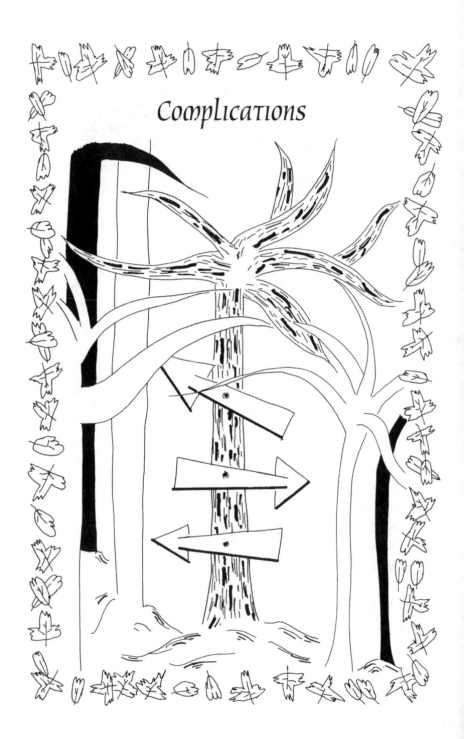

Now I See

by Joan Wolf

The realization was harsh. I remember the precise moment it hit. The sunlight was dancing through the window as I sat struggling to read an assigned chapter of a college textbook. As I read, my mind drifted back to a few years earlier, when reading print had not only been easy, but a pleasurable hobby.

But, sitting there on that sunny afternoon, trying to see through retinopathy-imposed blind spots, I think I understood for the first time that I would never again have the ability to read print smoothly.

I took off my glasses and let the sun warm my face. Realization sank in. From that moment on, I promised never again to take any part of my remaining eyesight for granted.

Naively, I once had thought myself beyond the reaches of diabetes. Denying the possibility of future problems with all the rebellious fervor I could muster, I acted as if I somehow had the power to ward off complications.

Inside this rebellion was the fear that I would not have the ability or strength to deal with complications, should they arise. I fell prey to the common misconception that blindness or neuropathy is somehow reserved for a few brave, strong individuals.

I knew that I could never face vision loss of any kind. I could never learn to live with diabetic complications or find the strength to carry on despite physical barriers. And, because of those feelings, I decided complications simply wouldn't happen to me.

Then, the day came. Retinopathy was diagnosed and an emotional flood was unleashed. The fabric of denial sewn together carefully throughout 15 years of diabetic life was torn into shreds. Something that was reserved for those brave, strong few had become part of my reality.

When retinopathy started affecting my eyesight, I began to grow more introspective. The vision of myself as one of those "handicapped" people confronted me.

I realized that I am no stronger or braver than I was before. I have not been changed in any grand, significant way because of retinopathy. I don't have genetically endowed strength that rises to the surface on diagnosis of diabetic complications. I have simply been forced into a position of no return—one of creative living. After years of being too afraid to look, I found that if I stepped aside from fear, I could find the strength in myself that I needed to deal with progressive vision loss.

Rather than seeing myself as different from those who do not have physical challenges, I began to realize how similar I am to everyone else in the world, whether they have diabetes or not. Each of us struggles in one way or another. Each of us laughs. Each of us cries. And all of us strive and stretch to live life to the fullest. I am no different in that respect from any other person.

Diabetes has taken things away from me, and it would be dishonest to deny the frustration I experience from living with inconvenience.

But diabetes has also given. It has taught me things I could not have learned through any other means. When the illusion of good health was stripped away, I was left with introspection, and I now have the ability to see within myself.

When I began to lose my sight, a sense we all prize as essential, I was forced to find other resources, those that lie deep beneath physical senses. There are talents, gifts, and skills that are just as essential as senses and they are beyond the physical reaches of diabetes.

Because what I thought would never happen is beginning to happen, I have learned precisely how much is possible in my life. I have developed a deeper sense of my own strength and a greater sense of inner peace. Each new challenge I overcome and each new obstacle I face proves that not only can I survive this disease, but that I can thrive.

At times, I have thought of diabetes as my most hated obstacle. But through all the anger, tears, and challenges, it has often proved to be my greatest asset; for, not only has it enabled me to reach essential parts of who I am, but it has given me the ability to touch who I wish to be.

Tell Me

by Linnea Mulder, RN

My friend and I were sitting together in the very first row, about 8 feet away from the panelists. We had already listened to some interesting topics—diabetes during adolescence, the impact of diabetes on families, and community resources, among others.

The next workshop, "The Psychosocial Issues of Diabetes," was the first to deal with complications. Four panelists (two men and two women) and a moderator participated.

The first panelist was in his late sixties and spoke of Charcot's joint, neuropathy, and the possible amputation of his foot. He was philosophical about a life well lived. The other panelists were in their late thirties and early forties and had lived with diabetes for 20 to 25 years.

One of the women related her experiences following her kidney transplant. The second man spoke about his feelings after recently having a fistula placed for dialysis. The last panelist to speak described her adjustment to living with severe vision loss due to retinopathy. I admired their ability to adapt and the strength of the human spirit when tested.

But my daughter is 6 years old. She was diagnosed when she was three, so she will have lived with diabetes for 20 years by the time she is a young woman. For now, please don't talk to me about vision loss, or dialysis, or Charcot's joint. The front row is closer than I want to be.

Instead, tell me how self-monitored blood glucose testing has improved our ability to control blood sugars. Tell me about the effectiveness of human insulin. Show me "user friendly," accurate glucose meters that a young child can use almost independently. Tell me about the potential for a non-invasive form of blood glucose monitoring. Tell me about the information that a glycated hemoglobin test offers. Help me. My daughter is too young, and I love her too much, to focus on anything else.

A break followed the panelists' discussion. My friend moved in her seat. Being good Scandinavians, neither one of us is prone to emotive speaking.

Our daughters have known each other since infancy. They have incorporated blood tests and insulin shots into their play along with bikes and Legos and crayons and Barbies. My friend said she couldn't talk about what we'd heard right then. That was good because neither could I.

Because of our daughters and their diabetes, we share a somewhat warped sense of humor and many support systems: friends, family, the diabetes team nurses, physicians, and dietitians—church members, school teachers, and our ADA-sponsored parent support group.

But it's still not easy. It wasn't easy in the early days to sit, trying to give a shot, on top of a squirming child while throwing Cheerios at a younger sister to keep her at bay. It's not easy as the reality slowly sinks in that diabetes never, not even once, takes a vacation, and that insulin, snack, and meal times are now permanently etched on whatever part of your brain that keeps track of those things. It's not easy to poke your child four or five times for a 2 a.m. blood sugar check, because the blood seems to have gone to sleep too. And how do you answer a child when she asks if her diabetes will be gone by her next birthday?

I am the one counting the losses, not my daughter. She doesn't remember a life without diabetes. Diabetes is certainly something that she can learn to live with. But it isn't easy, and I hope for more for her than that.

Yet, I am thankful for many things: my daughter's good health, her ability to adapt, and her stubborn independence (some of the time, anyway). I am thankful to live in an area where we have access to outstanding health professionals. I am thankful we have adequate health insurance.

But, most of all I am thankful for all the researchers whose dedication, time, effort, and hard work have given my daughter hope. I thank all of you who work to find ways to slow down or stop complications and to find a cure. I think of the ADA holiday "gift of hope" ornaments that we hang on our Christmas tree. Thank you researchers for this gift of hope, for this, in the end, is what keeps us going.

Editor's note: The results of the Diabetes Control and Complications Trial (DCCT) show that keeping blood glucose levels near normal does slow down or prevent 45 to 60% of diabetes-related complications.

Positively Angry About It All

by Susan Orzell

It's no secret that I love dogs. Will Rogers never met a man he didn't like, and I've never encountered a mutt that didn't delight me in some way. Except for one.

My friend, Ellen, owns an elderly apricot teacup poodle named, lamentably, Bitsey Ross, who has the intelligent little face, button nose, and the soft curly coat characteristic of the breed. Until recently, I detested the animal and never saw her without asking Ellen, "When are you going to do something about that dog?"

Bitsey Ross has diabetes. Every morning, Ellen gives her a shot of insulin and watches her carefully while she takes her exercise in the fenced yard. Some days, Bitsey laps bowls of ice cream, even though dairy products aren't good for canine systems, to compensate for low blood sugar.

The mechanics of caring for Bitsey Ross are no mystery to me. I've had type I diabetes for 17 years, and I understand all too well about balancing insulin, exercise, and diet to control the disease.

What I found baffling was why I had such an aversion to poor Bitsey. "When are you going to put her out of her misery?" I asked Ellen recently. "She's lost her eyesight. She has to be watched constantly. Why don't you do the kinder thing and...." to which Ellen responded calmly, "Why does your anger always surface whenever you see my dog?"

She was right, of course. The problem was not the diabetic poodle and certainly not envy at Ellen's willingness to adapt to her difficulties. The issue was that, as much as I believed that I had long since struggled through a lengthy denial stage and had fully accepted my own diabetes, something in Bitsey's condition and her resulting vulnerability caused undeniable rage to roil up inside me.

Upon introspection, it horrified me to realize that if I controlled the fate of Bitsey Ross, I would have her humanely euthanized. Yes, it is because she, like me, is insulin-dependent and spends her days balancing on a tightwire from which she, too, occasionally topples.

I know that anger can be a positive emotion. It can be energizing and motivating. Angry people who direct their outrage into positive channels can accomplish a great deal. A person with diabetes who takes charge of his or her anger can use it to focus on controlling the condition. It's the old, "This dratted thing isn't going to beat me!" syndrome.

The real problems start when the natural feeling of anger is denied, usually by someone who considers it an impolite, unacceptable, and ungovernable emotion. Buried in the subconscious, it then emerges in some disguised form. Often, it masquerades as depression.

I'm sure Bitsey Ross never philosophizes about her condition. She goes about her life with unabashed enthusiasm. "She's French," Ellen explains.

"She's pathetically uneducated about self-care, but at least she's not preoccupied with it," I add.

Even her blindness seems inconsequential, as she draws on her other senses and her trust in the humans in her life to enjoy what each day brings. She knows immediately when I walk through the door, alerted by my scent and that of my own dogs that clings to me, and is delighted by my visit. I'm the one who struggles against her condition, irritated by the way it forces me to face the possibilities inherent in the disease we share.

That's another reason I'm angry at poor innocent Bitsey: I resent the way she makes ignoring the possibility of complications impossible.

I might add, though, that the last time I held the improbably tiny dog on my lap, stroked her silky ears, and mused about her unseeing eyes, I made a mental note to check my daybook for the date of my next visit to my ophthalmologist. "Now there's an example of positive transference," I told Ellen.

Should I develop severe retinopathy as a result of diabetes, there's a good chance my sight can be saved with timely laser surgery, an option not open to our canine counterparts. The trick is to be aware enough of the nasty capacities of the disease to forestall problems before they occur. Bitsey's unwitting, mute testimony is a nudge in that direction.

The memorable lessons are often taught by the strangest teachers, aren't they?

PARKING LOT LIBERATION

by Leslie Dawson

I stood beside a battered blue Buick in the parking lot, waiting for the bank to open at 9 a.m. "I have to transfer some money before I go to work," I told the man sitting in the Buick. "We made a $60 mistake in balancing somewhere."

"Yeah," he responded. "I gotta make a deposit, then go pay my dentist, and then I'm due for a dialysis treatment at noon."

"Dialysis? You're on kidney dialysis?" I exclaimed.

"Yeah. Three times a week."

I took a good look at him. He was a slender, short black man. He looked healthy, with a few grey strands in his black hair. He had a thin mustache, and wore a green knit shirt, and on his right ring finger, a gold insignia ring. Altogether, he had a sporty look.

"Do you have diabetes?" I enquired further.

"No. I got kidney disease from high blood pressure."

I was stunned. I have had a morbid fear of kidney disease and dialysis all my diabetic life.

"How long have you been on dialysis?" I asked. Was it one year, or maybe two?

"Oh, 12 years, off and on. I had a transplant for about 8 years before I rejected it. I'm on dialysis now, but I'm on the transplant list again."

He leaned back from his car's steering wheel. He looked relaxed, even content. How could that be?

"Look...I have diabetes, and kidney disease is my worst nightmare." I felt my voice tremble slightly. It was a little embarrassing, but I'd never met a kidney patient before. I hungered for information from a real person, not just a magazine article. "Would you tell me about it? I mean...."

"Sure, miss," he said. "It's not bad really, not as bad as people make out. The people who have problems are the ones that don't do what they're told...they don't come in for dialysis all the time, or take their medication."

"The main problem is gettin' tired," he said. "Just wipes some people out for a whole day. For others, it's not so bad."

It's not so bad, I thought with disbelief. Lying for hours, with a machine cleaning your blood. Totally dependent on a system of tubes and filters sucking wastes from your body.

"What about the itch?" I persisted. I'd heard that was unbearable.

"Oh, when it's itchy, it's because some minerals are missing—phosphorus, and some others I can't remember. They have medications that really work. And some creams. You just have to take the medications, that's all."

"What's your name, please? I'm Leslie." Suddenly I remembered my manners.

"Tim," he said. "You know I worked full time for the first 10 years I was on dialysis. Ten-hour shifts 4 days a week. Then the fatigue got to me and I quit. But you know, I lead a pretty normal life."

He told me that his medical team tried to persuade him to use a portable device, something like an insulin pump. He'd decided against it, for various reasons, but it worked for others.

There had to be some horrors, I thought. "What about dietary restrictions? I hear you can't eat much protein."

"Well, there're some restrictions. Meat and dairy products and such. But I've experimented a bit, and there're some foods I still eat that I shouldn't, but I just don't eat as much. Doesn't seem to bother me."

He looked up, then down at his watch. "Hey...3 minutes until opening time."

People had lined up at the bank door. Tim got out of his car and we walked together to the sidewalk.

"Tim, thank you. God, you don't know what you've done for me. Sometimes I get obsessed with my diabetes. I smell ketones in my urine for a few days and I tell myself I've just got 5 years to live. And I've sworn that when my kidneys go, and I have to be on dialysis, I'll just shoot myself. I mean, seriously."

Tim stopped walking. He turned and looked at me. Seriously. He took my hands in his, bowed his head, and quietly prayed for my good health. People in the bank line moved past us, politely ignoring the strange duo at the bank door.

I used my sleeve to blot the tears streaming down my face. We said goodbye. I went into the lobby and transferred money from savings to checking. I don't even remember seeing Tim after that. I do remember, on my way to work, my feet felt light as I walked. A smile played across my face as the traffic whizzed by in the September sun.

The Driver's Seat

The light seemed unbearable as I stepped outside the
doctor's office. The dark glasses the retinologist gave
me to shield my dilated eyes from the sunlight also hid the
tears that began to flow now that I was alone.

No person with diabetes likes to hear about the complications he or she might face because of the disease. I had
read the reports. Diabetes was a leading cause of blindness
in the United States. But years ago I pushed that possibility
to the back of my mind. Reality, however, had finally hit.
One day 3 years ago, I saw a reddish film of blood in my
left eye, and more than 30 years of denial dissolved in a
moment, leaving me an emotional mess.

The retinologist confirmed my worst fears. He told me
my left eye had hemorrhaged and was seriously affected
with advanced proliferative retinopathy. I had a less-serious
condition called background retinopathy in my right eye
and retinal detachment in both. I would need immediate
laser treatments and a possible vitrectomy, an operation that
replaces damaged eye fluid. It would be a difficult year.

Thank God I had a wonderful support group of family
and friends, and the team of counselors and educators at a
newly opened diabetes management and research center in
Los Angeles. I started attending a therapy group for people
with diabetes and unloaded a lot of anxiety, guilt, and fears
with others who faced similar problems.

I concentrated harder on my work. I found solace in my religious beliefs and prayed I would not need the operation. But with each laser session, it became clear that an operation was inevitable. After 11 treatments and almost 10,000 individual "blasts" of the laser beam, my retinologist and I set the date for the vitrectomy.

By then I was totally prepared, physically, mentally, and spiritually.

In the examining room the day before the operation, my diabetes specialist asked how I was doing and whether I was anxious about the upcoming procedure. I remember his surprise when I told him how good I felt and that I was completely confident things would be all right.

My operation was a success, and with each check-up, my retinologist marveled at my recovery. I was his "miracle patient." It's been almost 3 years since the operation, and my vision is 20/20 in both eyes.

So what was different about my case? Certainly the prognosis wasn't very good when the retinopathy was diagnosed. What happened to turn my situation around?

A wonderful surgeon? Yes. Modern laser technology? That, too. A great support group? Of course. But another important thing was something I did myself. I changed my thinking.

I decided to take control. I was not going to let the disease control me. I stopped calling myself a "diabetic"; I was a person with diabetes. I wasn't going to just "cope" with complications; I intended to take charge of my diabetes and my entire life. I relaxed and transformed the anxiety and worry to peace and strength.

Perhaps if the operation had gone differently, I would have a different attitude. But I don't think so. I had prepared myself for whatever the outcome might be, and that included losing my sight. My situation wasn't special and I wasn't simply unlucky. In fact, luck had nothing to do with it.

I had lived a life of uncontrolled diabetes, and it was inevitable that my body should develop this complication. Certainly, if I drive 100 miles an hour straight toward a brick wall, I expect to crash. But I won't hit the wall if I slow up and turn the wheel. And that's what I did.

I am not deluding myself that I'm now free of other complications. Living with diabetes is not easy, but my attitude is completely different, and that's what really matters.

I know the truth; I'm in the driver's seat, and I can control this thing.

Five Decades

by Daniel B. Dallas

1956: I'm an assistant editor on the staff of an engineering magazine, where the work is demanding but sedentary. I'm 20 pounds overweight, have no interest in exercise, and smoke relentlessly.

I'm also trying to ignore a problem: recurring chest pains. A friend insists that I seek medical attention. Thus begins my long association with Dr. Eugene Steinberger, who hospitalizes me immediately. But I'll be OK—I'm only 36, and nothing bad happens to people that young.

I'm lying in a hospital bed, enjoying a cigarette, when the heart attack hits. It's a big one—it hits with the crushing force of a linebacker.

I'm in the hospital for five weeks. When I'm discharged, Dr. Steinberger tells me to stop smoking and develop a different lifestyle. I tell him I'll take his suggestions under advisement. I go home, and right back to three packs a day.

So my father died of a coronary at 52. I'll be OK. And anyway, I catch Dr. Steinberger in the act of hiding his pipe during an office visit. Physician, heal thyself!

1965: I'm attending a trade show in Philadelphia when the second heart attack hits. The pain is incredible. They fly me back to Detroit, and I wind up in the same hospital, and almost in the same bed. This time I go home after three weeks. I'm given a strict injunction to stop smoking and begin dieting.

But I refuse. I will not change my lifestyle! And don't think I'm being dumb. I couldn't be dumb. I'm now senior associate editor.

1972: I'm in Philadelphia again, at a seminar. It's not terribly interesting, but as executive editor, I'm obliged to attend. There's plenty of ice water at my table, and it is, without a doubt, the best water I've ever tasted. I've drunk half a pitcher and have gone to the restroom five times before it occurs to me that something is terribly wrong.

Two days later, I'm in Dr. Steinberger's office. He orders me to the hospital immediately. They run tests, and I'm told I'm "dumping sugar."

Whatever dumping sugar means, it couldn't be too bad; my weight is dropping precipitously. That's good, isn't it?

Dr. Steinberger tells me my glucose reading is over 400. "Four hundred out of what?" I ask. He doesn't smile.

I'm discharged within a week. I'm now taking something called Diabinese.

1980: I have a persistent case of laryngitis. Dr. Steinberger refers me to a throat specialist, who asks if I smoke. "Yes, I do, three packs a day," I admit, shamefaced. He gives me a choice: Quit smoking or quit talking.

I flush with anger. With a flourish, I take a pack of cigarettes out of my shirt pocket and hurl it into the doctor's wastebasket. He's impressed by my dramatic actions, but questions whether I will be able to make it home without stopping off to buy another pack. I tell him I will, and I mean it. I know I will never smoke again.

I am 60 years of age, and I calculate that I have smoked at least 850,000 cigarettes to date. How many acres of tobacco is that? How many bales? How many quarts of nicotinic acid?

Why does it take so long to get smart?

1993: I'm 11 years retired from my post as editorial director. My weight is 165—down from the 192 I carried in the salad days of my disbelief. My glucose, faithfully tested each morning, stays in a range comfortably below 140 mg/dl. I do five miles a day on my aerobic bicycle and take my insulin regularly. I am, by every criterion, an ideal medical patient.

An ideal patient who owes his life to heart bypass surgery in 1983. An ideal patient, functioning on half a heart.

The great and abiding puzzle is this: If I can face reality without flinching today, at 73, why couldn't I face it back in my 30s? What was the nature of that cloud-cover that blanketed my mind so completely? What was it that led me to waste so many valuable years that could have been used to make myself healthier?

Dr. Steinberger—frail, aged, gentle, diabetic, and neuropathic—assures me that I'm not unusual. I'm merely typical of a certain type of patient. Some patients, he says, refuse to learn from their medical history and are condemned to repeat it.

Few of those repeaters are as lucky as I.

I'm alive.

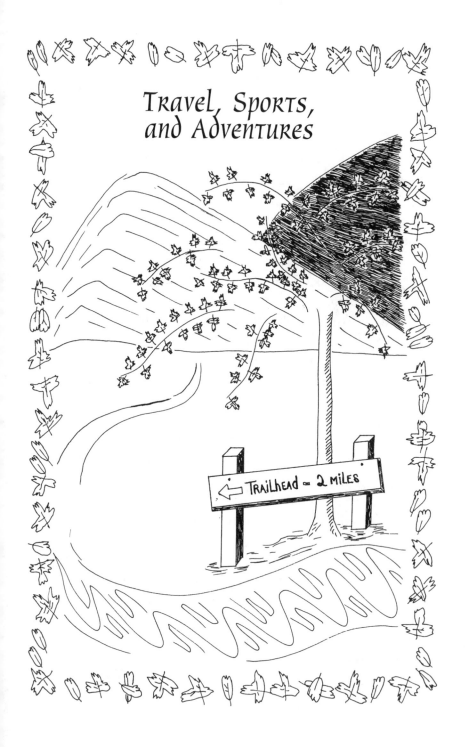

Travel, Sports, and Adventures

TRAILHEAD ← 2 MILES

At Home on the Range

by Jackie A. Holmgren

A little over 100 years ago, I wouldn't have been here herding cows from the back of a horse. Number one, I'm a woman. Number two, I have type I diabetes. That would have cut my life short, male or female!

My husband and I lease a large cow outfit in the Missouri Breaks of Montana and punch cattle on it. Our ranch is surrounded by reminders of the past: a grave of a man killed by Indians; two early forts that offered protection to the trappers, settlers, and the steamboats that came up the Missouri River; and an old saloon just over the hill at the mouth of Dog Creek where early-day cowboys had hell-raisin' times. This was where hundreds of thousands of cattle were pushed north across the Missouri to fresh range in the Milk River country.

Even today, the only way to get around our ranch is on horseback, in all types of weather, fording the Judith River that bisects our ranch. We cannot eat or even sleep according to nature's plan for gentler folks.

Eight years ago, I was on an elk hunting trip in the Beartooth Mountains. I had to keep getting out of my tent at night, despite a howling snowstorm, to relieve myself. I was so thirsty I kept a canteen of water in my bedroll so it wouldn't freeze. If I had been in the Sahara Desert, instead of the frozen, Montana mountain country, I couldn't have felt thirstier.

The only thing that saved me from ketoacidosis, I believe, was all the exercise I got trucking up and down mountainsides and cutting piles of wood for the fire. When we rode back into town, I went to see the saw-bones.

Then I was glad it was 1983 instead of 1883. I didn't go to the hospital, but I took a week-long course in diabetes management. I got myself one of those new-fangled blood glucose meters, and I started giving myself shots.

I read books on diabetes management and came across one that described how to mimic the action of a normal pancreas with multiple injections.

My lifestyle, you see, just didn't fit the timetable that my diabetes routine dictated. I didn't want to give up any of my cowgirl life, so with my doctor's approval, I switched to multiple injections. I felt as though I had been released from the crow-bar motel! My blood sugar normalized, and I realized that I could rein in the diabetes and retake control of my life.

I am still where I love to be, out in the big sky country. And big sky country in my family means cattle, horses, and range. The things I do daily take me far from home and modern civilization. Horses and cows have changed little since the 1870s.

Every spring we gather all the mother cows off the windswept winter range and put them in large pastures to calve. We ride these pastures everyday to make sure all is going well. March in Montana is not really spring and in snow and cold the little calves are born.

After calving comes branding. All of the family and friends come to help, so branding becomes a social, as well as hard-working, time of the year.

In summer, we drive the cows and calves to new pastures. We ride out to find strays and to help any sick critters. This can get pretty exciting in tough country, when my horse is going lickety-split after a doggie who sure doesn't act sick! With ropes twirling, we "head and heel" the animal. Then we can give a shot or a pill.

In the fall we gather again to round up the cattle and count them. It takes many rides to dig them all out of the hills. The calves are weaned from their mothers and shipped to town. The cows are put out to winter pasture, so they can be fed in bad weather. We use a team of draft horses and a pickup. It sometimes takes all day to get them fed in a Montana blizzard. By spring the cycle begins again.

We break our own horses. My husband can "ride anything with hair" as they say of bronco twisters, and I can hold my own. It takes a string of six horses for each of us to keep from being "footback." Most days we ride more than 15 miles.

Cowgirl or not, I still have to pack my meter, strips, and a meal along in my saddle bags. I go to the doctor "pretty regular." My glycated hemoglobin level (A_{1c}) is normal and I have had no complications. I try to eat my good, lean beef with complex carbohydrates, and every now and then I even have a piece of pie at the family gatherings.

I guess my point is that even though I live my life happy in the freewheelin' style of the past, the present and future are mine because of modern medical advances.

Editor's note: Exercise is not recommended to treat diabetic ketoacidosis (DKA). See a physician immediately if you suspect that you or a loved one might be experiencing DKA.

Grand Canyon Sweet

by Tullia Limarzi

A s we climbed into our car for the 10-minute drive to the trailhead, I cried, both from joy and from anticipation. Fifteen months before, just diagnosed with non-insulin-dependent (type II) diabetes, my middle-aged, overweight self had trouble walking briskly one whole turn around the quarter-mile track at our local high school. Now I dared to tackle the Grand Canyon.

I'd read everything I could get my hands on about the Canyon. I learned that it could be a treacherous place as well as an enchanting place and that aerobic fitness was essential for walking and hiking safely through its changing elevations.

Could I make it? I had my doubts. After all, I had been sedentary. I had been through yo-yo weight gains and losses until diabetes made me realize I had to exercise and control my eating now—no more maybes or tomorrows.

But then again, I also had reason to be confident. Since beginning my diabetic diet, I had lost 30 pounds and, perhaps more importantly, had exercised faithfully. By walking and using a cross-country ski machine, I had maintained a regimen of aerobic workouts at least four times a week.

My husband and I had decided to make our first day at the Canyon a trial of our abilities (even he wasn't sure of his capabilities in a strange environment). We live in New

York City and had done some hiking and camping in the Appalachian Mountains, but we had never experienced high-altitude hiking or desert conditions, both of which occur within the Grand Canyon.

We would first try a short, yet strenuous hike, 3 miles round trip, with a 1,500-foot elevation change. As promised in our guidebook, we got marvelous open views of the Canyon, and we completed the hike in less time than the three hours the guidebook allowed.

We spent the next day exploring the rim by foot and shuttle bus. We moved at our own pace: stopping to stare down into an eerie abyss that plunges 1,000 feet, scanning a distant plateau for abandoned mining camps, or simply gazing in wonderment at chasm and sky.

By our third day, we were ready to experience the 12-mile round trip along the popular Bright Angel Trail, a path first carved by Indians, now used by hikers and mule trains to travel to and from the Colorado River.

Our route would take us 9 miles down, then 3,200 feet up to Indian Gardens, an oasis where we'd find water and shade. Then we'd have a 3-mile side trip to get a bird's-eye view of the Colorado River at Plateau Point. The side trip meant walking under a relentless sun through desert where the temperature was 100°F. Our hike was not a mere physical test; our exertion was the means for taking in the Canyon's natural beauty and splendor.

Once again we set off at dawn, and almost immediately we came face to face with a lone bighorn sheep who had left the canyon's precipitous slopes to descend the winding trail with us. Later, in the desert, we watched a collared lizard slither across sun-parched clay and scrub.

Throughout the day we stopped to relish the Canyon's innumerable crests and gorges.

And thanks to our fellow travelers from around the world, my husband and I did more than just savor one of the Earth's natural wonders. We experienced a communal adventure unlike any other we had ever known. We doused our sweltering heads and filled our canteens with water alongside an Australian family and Italian students, and we shared lunch in a log shelter with a Danish couple. In spite of our cultural and political differences, we shared the Canyon's challenges and delights as members of the human family.

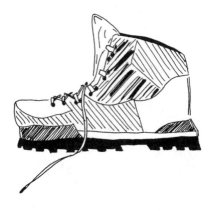

By the end of the day, the climb back to the rim had challenged my physical endurance to the limit: I had worked aerobically for four and a half hours. I ended my adventure exhausted and exhilarated. I would never ask to have diabetes, but since I do have it, I'm glad it motivated me to get into shape. I had not known how emotionally uplifting fitness can be.

Riding High in Middle Age

by John Royer

In August of 1989, my friend Bob convinced me to buy a mountain bike. I was skeptical.

I told the bike salesman that I weighed 250 pounds, had high blood pressure, had recently quit smoking, and wanted to try exercise because I hated the diet my doctor gave me. The salesman chuckled and said he had a bike for me.

I went home a few hundred dollars poorer with a first class mountain bike. I was 43 years old with a wife and three children, and I wanted to be healthy.

Mild hills that were no trouble for me to walk were gargantuan to bike. The 18 gears were not enough, and I struggled to go even short distances. My bike seat, a special gel-filled model, felt as hard as a rock, and my thighs ached. Misery was my daily riding companion.

So, I ate to keep up my strength. And my morale. Perhaps biking was a bad idea; the money was wasted; I was a fool. Food became more important than ever.

Eventually, Bob suggested I try an every-other-day training schedule to give my muscles time to rest and rebuild. It worked. I felt better, and I lost 10 pounds, even though I was overeating. The salesman and my doctor had told me I had to exercise *and* diet. They were wrong I thought. I was up to 4 miles.

Winter set in, and it was cold, too cold to bike. My weight came back, and I let it. "At least," I thought, "my legs are stronger," while I rounded off my winter diet with peanut butter crackers and whole milk at bedtime.

Spring 1990 came, and the bike came out of the garage. Pain came with it. To my horror, my hard-earned muscle had slipped away during a winter of lethargy and overeating. In a few diligent weeks, however, it returned, and I aimed for 10 miles!

I lost 5 pounds and stuck at 245. I rode harder but ate more. Then I was laid up for a week with severe intestinal pain and a high fever.

Eventually, I was riding 10 to 20 miles a day. My weight stayed the same, but my waist was shrinking. My wife bought me a cold weather biking outfit. Extra-large, of course.

Winter struck, and the bike got parked. In January 1991, the intestinal ailment returned. I ended up in the emergency room. There I admitted to the doctor that since mid-December, I had experienced dry mouth and excessive urination. Plus, I was dropping 2 to 3 pounds a day and had lost 10 pounds in four days.

With test results in hand, he identified the cause of some of my problems—type II diabetes caused by over-40, overweight conditions. He grinned and said that I could certainly stand to lose some weight but not this way. He was a remarkably witty fellow.

Numerous tests at my doctor's office showed that my pancreas was on strike and a spastic intestine had caused the fever. He sent me to a dietitian with stern instructions to take her dietary advice seriously. I had not followed his typed instructions, he said, so maybe counseling from a professional would work.

A very kind lady with enormous patience explained how to get the fat and sugar out of my diet by eating lots of fruit, cutting down serving sizes, figuring food exchanges, and setting regular meal times. She said periodic food binges could be worked into my plan. I was amazed.

The doctor's diet sheet may have said this, but not as eloquently. And I could ask questions! It sounded easy.

It turned out to be easy. Wonder of wonders!

I followed my diet with a vengeance. Without it, I had two alternatives: pills to encourage my pancreas to produce insulin (added to the two I was taking for high blood pressure) or insulin injections—reasons enough to stay on my diet!

Spring came and I attacked the roadways again. On a 94° day in July 1991, I rode a record 45 miles. I weighed 210 pounds, and my only complaint was a sore derriere.

My blood pressure is now down to 140/80, I'm off the diuretic, and my blood pressure medication has been cut by half. My blood glucose is in the 90 to 110 mg/dl range. I've learned that careful monitoring of food and drink combined with exercise can produce some rather wonderful results.

My weight and my health are excellent. I have conquered smoking, obesity, high blood pressure, and adult diabetes in middle age, and I am enjoying this life. It's the only one I've got!

All the News That's Fit to Print

by Alfred R. Evans

When my doctor told me I had type II diabetes, I was devastated!

My health problems had actually begun about a month before. I was putting out four weekly publications on deadline. I was also meeting payroll and other expenses and dealing with the stress of selling my small corporation.

On Father's Day, I was carrying lawn chairs off the deck of our home when it collapsed under me. I wasn't hurt, but the shock plus the business stress apparently helped trigger the diabetes.

A week later I found myself getting very thirsty and getting up three or four times a night. One evening I sat down to watch a favorite TV show, and the screen blurred before my eyes. Another week passed, and I noticed I was losing weight.

I made an appointment with my doctor for several days later. My wife felt I should see him sooner and moved the appointment up. It turned out, according to my physician, that if I had waited one more day, I would have wound up in a coma.

My doctor ordered me to the hospital. Soon after I checked in, the nurses began loading me up with insulin. In the next four days, I learned new ways to take care of myself: Take shots, watch my diet, and get rid of stress. They showed me videotapes about other people with diabetes who were successfully managing it.

I was released from the hospital in time to sign the papers that made the sale of my business official. That ended some of the stress. The very next week I began reading everything I could about diabetes treatment. One very helpful book, found by my local librarian, addressed reversing type II diabetes. Although at that time neither my doctor nor I thought that was possible, I enthusiastically began to diet and exercise to improve my health.

My wife, Eileen, continued working for the firm that had purchased our newspapers, so I became a motivated house husband. I purchased several cookbooks printed especially for people with diabetes and began cooking for my wife, our three children still living at home, and myself. I also did the shopping and other household chores. The entire family started eating better. A teenage daughter lost 30 pounds, and a sports-minded son found he had more stamina.

In our town we have a community center with basketball courts, a running and walking track, a weight room, and exercise equipment. We purchased a family membership, and I began a program to get—and keep—in shape. I would pack up my sweats and basketball, go over to the center, shoot baskets for an hour, then ride an exercise bike for 15 or 20 minutes, weigh myself, take a shower, and head for home. When warm weather arrived, my family and I took bike rides, shot baskets in our driveway, and began to swim regularly.

A few months later, I noticed my afternoon blood sugar readings were dropping. I would sometimes have a reading as low as 59 before taking my evening shot. That seemed very low to my doctor and me, so one night, with his approval, I skipped the insulin. I checked my blood sugar two more times that evening and early the next morning. All the readings were still in the 80 to 120 mg/dl range.

On my next visit to my doctor, he noted that because of my strict diet and exercise, my need for insulin was diminishing. He asked me to drop it two units a week, check the readings, and then give his office a call. The readings remained in the normal range. In a few weeks, I was completely off the insulin. I have now gone three years with normal readings.

I have become a newspaper consultant for publishers of hometown weekly newspapers. I want to help these papers survive. Besides, we have 14 children...and of the 11 out of school, 10 have been or are in the newspaper and printing trade. One even ran a typesetter to earn her way through college. Our remaining two boys at home also want to learn the newspaper and printing trade.

I still check my blood sugar every other day. I can't believe I am not taking any shots. I still watch my diet and am sure to exercise faithfully. I may be one of the lucky ones, but if I should stray, I am sure I would be back on insulin within a short while. I feel better now than I have for years, and I'd like to keep it that way.

Out on The Ice

by Carl F. Crumpton

I began ice fishing with my son, Paul, a few years ago. Although he showed me how to hold the rod, I soon learned that my hands and fingers were not as sensitive as they should be for feeling the ever-so-light movement of a crappie taking the lure into its mouth.

That's because I have type II diabetes, and I no longer have a delicate sense of feel in my old hands. With the cold making heavily insulated gloves necessary, I seldom felt any sign of a biting crappie. Paul caught lots of fish, but I didn't.

He suggested the use of a small Styrofoam bobber so I could see the movement that I couldn't feel. He rigged my line with such a bobber. It worked. I could see the bobber move ever so slightly and could set the hook in time. Soon, I, too, began catching those lightly nibbling crappie. Since then, I have used a bobber in many of my fishing endeavors but especially when fishing for crappie or white bass through the ice. My success has led to a new nick-name, too.

I was fishing alone in early January 1991 and having fair luck catching crappie. Two gentlemen walked out onto the ice about 200 yards away. They fished at some distance from me, so I was startled to look up and see them standing nearby, watching. When I said hello, one of them said, "Don't mind us, we're novices at this and want to see how it's done. We haven't even had a bite and were heading home. You have several nice crappie in your bucket, and we want to watch you for a few minutes."

I said, "Try those holes near where you're standing. Get your crappie jigs down to 12 feet. I'm using brown and orange tube lures, but other colors may work as well or better."

They followed my suggestions and soon both were catching fish. They did a mighty good job!

We met on the ice again a few days later. They stopped to see how I was doing and to thank me for showing them where and how to fish through the ice. "We were thrilled to catch the fish, but we both also enjoyed watching how you worked those bobbers and landed your fish," one said.

"It's clumsy, but it works for me," I replied.

Twelve feet of line is too long for me to lift a fish out onto the ice with the rod alone. With the bobber on the line, I cannot reel it in, so I must first set the hook with the rod and then take the line with my other hand and continue pulling the fish up. I lay the rod down and bring the fish out onto the ice with a hand-over-hand motion.

"We think it's beautiful the way you land those fish. We've told lots of people about your technique and your success using it. I hope you don't mind," one of them said, "but I have dubbed you the bobber man."

I didn't mind at all. In fact, I sort of liked the ring of it. When the gentlemen went on their way, I reflected on the new nickname and my diabetes. A simple adjustment to my condition had given me great success. During the first three weeks of January 1991, I caught 120 pounds of crappie that I shared with family and friends and froze for later use. On two different occasions, I got my limit of 50 fish in about two hours. The bobber man? It fits. I don't mind that nickname at all.

And I like what ice fishing has done for me. Walking long distances on the ice and drilling holes through it provides exercise that burns calories and helps keep my blood sugar in the proper range. Just keeping myself warm when the wind chill is as low as -30°F uses a lot of calories.

Being away from the house for several hours at a time reduces the number of trips I might otherwise make to the fridge. Jigging, watching that bobber, and landing the fish are relaxing—and also help control my blood sugar. Diabetes makes ice fishing tougher for me, but ice fishing helps control my diabetes.

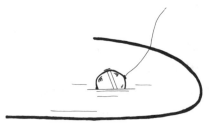

The fish I catch provide good protein. With side dishes of homemade whole grain bread, oyster mushrooms, mixed vegetables, and a bit of fruit, I have a great meal to help control my blood glucose levels.

Sometimes I broil the fish, other times I fry them in a little canola oil. Before frying, I coat the fillets with my specially seasoned pancake flour to which I add miller's bran for extra roughage. Daughter Sheryl thinks it is the greatest way to prepare fish and asks me to always fry an extra large batch so she can take the excess home to be enjoyed as part of her future meals—compliments of good ol' Dad, the bobber man.

Peak Experiences

by Leslie Trent Conger

I looked at my husband, Alan, and asked the inevitable question, "Why do we *do* these things?"

We were ascending Huron Peak, one of Colorado's "14ers," or mountains with summits exceeding 14,000 feet. We were making our ascent in the usual way: tired from lack of sleep the night before and feeling like work horses. The packs on our backs were heavy with food, water, and extra clothing. It was hard to believe we were doing this of our own volition.

Climbing 14ers is demanding in every way, from the physically arduous work of hiking several miles and gaining 3,000 to 5,000 feet of elevation, to negotiating the varied characteristics of the mountain peaks where the Colorado weather can suddenly become wild and unpredictable. You're exposed to the elements once you leave timberline at about 11,500 feet, and you face the dangers of unstable rock scrambling and slipping on dry, dusty soil at steep inclines. Then there's the fear of falling you must cope with as you ascend precarious boulders. At any time, you could turn your ankle or lose sight of your trail and wind up wandering in the wilderness.

I started hiking 14ers in 1986, 6 months before I was diagnosed with type I diabetes. I hated hiking at first. It was hard work and I didn't like how I felt on top— exhausted and disheveled. I remember thinking to myself,

"Never again! I don't think my body can handle this!" But Alan enjoyed the climbs and we had friends who also enjoyed them.

Not being one to let them go without me, I was compelled to try it again. Suddenly, on my third climb, I developed what we know in Colorado as "Fourteener Fever." Something about the particular mountain, coupled with the company of good friends, turned me into a glutton for punishment! Of the 54 peaks in Colorado that are 14,000 feet or more, I've now ascended 24.

Hiking these mountains with diabetes is quite daring. The fine balance between insulin and food intake is a daily challenge for all of us with diabetes, but even more so in this extreme situation. I check my blood sugar every hour—no picnic in cold, windy conditions! Sometimes I have to eat more than I want, just to keep my sugars "beefed up" for the demands of the hike.

One of my 14er friends, Dewi (pronounced "Davie"), has lupus. She can't get too much sun, so she hikes in long pants, a long-sleeved shirt, a hat to shield her face, and lots of sunscreen. We both hike at a moderate pace so as not to tax our bodies too much. And we both experience consequences after a climb: She has significant pain in her joints for days afterward, and I, along with a crippling build-up of lactic acid in my muscles, can experience low blood sugar for a couple of days while my body replenishes its electrolytes.

Recently, when Dewi and I pondered why we subject ourselves to these ordeals, we agreed that on some level, it's plain foolish to put ourselves in this kind of jeopardy. But almost in the same breath, we talked excitedly and joyfully about what motivates us to hike 14ers.

The peaks themselves are awesome—majestic and wild barrenness on a grand scale—yet featuring intricate, delicate life and other subtle characteristics. And I am always amazed at the progress made simply by putting one foot in front of another. A distant summit can appear to be unattainable, then all of a sudden it's reached.

Hiking is also a wonderful way to enjoy friendship. The toughness of a climb can bond people together in the same way any life circumstance does that requires caring and character from its participants.

Finally, there is no feeling like reaching a summit, even if the climb has been utterly fatiguing, frustrating, or frightening. Signing my name on the register, taking in the panoramic view of neighboring distant peaks, and knowing that I did it in spite of physical limitation sends me even higher emotionally.

We are more than just bodies forced to live with self-denial because of a disease. We have something inside of us that yearns for more. I am no hotshot athlete. I am, however, a person who desires to get the very most from life, in spite of having diabetes. All it takes is some planning: I stay in shape all year and take the precautions necessary to ensure that my 14er experiences are safe and enjoyable.

Why do we do these things?

Because we *love* doing them!

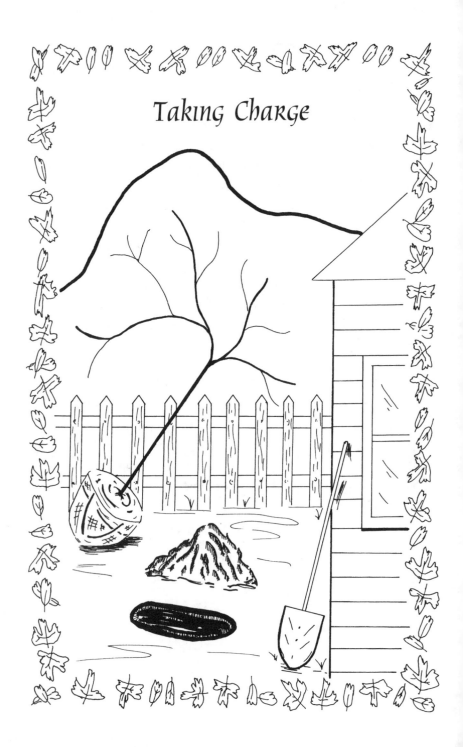

Taking Charge

I'm no Fred Astaire

by Susan L. Hildebrandt

Most of the time, I feel like Fred Astaire. It may look easy to live with diabetes, but it's a lot of hard work behind the scenes.

If someone asks me what it's like to live with diabetes, I laugh. To the uninitiated, the daily regimen of blood testing, insulin juggling, exchanges, and exercise is mind-boggling. They don't know, and I can't tell them, how many steps there are in this dance. Diabetes sneakily affects virtually all aspects of my life.

I got insulin-dependent diabetes at age 25. I am 31 now, and strangely enough, I only vaguely remember what my life was like before the choreography got so complicated. (What person with diabetes doesn't automatically convert Haagen-Dazs into exchanges?)

Getting diabetes in my mid-twenties was both devastating and well-timed. At that age, I could think of myself as a "person" with diabetes, but what made it particularly hard was how long it took me to gain some control. I was an avid exerciser and oat bran devotee, pre-diabetes. Well sure, I thought, I just have to eat right, work out, take a little insulin (snap my fingers, click my heels), and I'll be fine. None of those nasty complications for me in the future.

But that didn't happen. My blood sugars shot up high, then swooped down. I got depressed. I felt very, very old and sick, and I took more and more shots daily. My only cheery memories of those first few years are from my "honeymoon period," which lasted an unbelievable 12 months.

Unfortunately, the honeymoon had to end. Frustrated with the jerky rhythms of the three-shot-a-day routine, I turned to the insulin pump. With scenes from the Bionic Woman in my head and the gloomy belief that I would never wear a bikini again, I decided to give it a try.

It certainly wasn't love at first sight. It was hard to convince myself that wearing a needle in my stomach was a wonderful and enviable thing. And the plastic paraphernalia that came with the pump kindled no spark of joy within either.

The pump opened up a whole new world for me, however, in the lingerie department. For instance, how to wear an object the size of a deck of cards somewhere in my clothing where it wouldn't be mistaken for a walkie-talkie? Excuse me, lady, your beeper seems to have fallen into your pantyhose. Luckily for me, panty girdles hadn't gone the way of 1950s movies, but many saleswomen questioned my need for tummy flattening panels in a size 6.

Then there were the delicately phrased locker-room questions. Not needing any insulin while I am exercising, I would put the pump in my purse and allow the tubing to swish behind me. There were tactful comments about how I seemed to have gotten something stuck to myself in the shower (a common occurrence, I know). And subtle, sensitive questions like, "What in God's name is that in your stomach?"

Using a blood glucose monitor also requires a steely nerve. There was the time I was nearly arrested in the U.S.

Senate visitors' gallery. Working late one evening, I reck-lessly pulled out my meter to check my blood sugar. Vigilant security agents thought I had sneaked in a tape recorder.

Pleading that I had diabetes, I endured long minutes of hissed reprimands as the agent interrogated me. I tried to ignore the bevy of security agents, complete with ear-phones, who had promptly appeared to monitor my suspi-cious behavior.

Years later, my machines continue to set the tempo for my waltz with diabetes. I still don't have perfect control. My blood sugars frequently look like temperature readings on Mars, but the pump has given me flexibility and a more normal life.

The diabetes is better, too. I don't spend time thinking about complications so much as I worry about the fat con-tent of cashews and the amount of insulin I'll need to cover a late dinner out. I could never have reached this point without the support—which falls somewhere between breezy acceptance and total frustration—of my husband and family.

I keep abreast of the latest research (if I can under-stand it), hit the exercise club, eat three square meals a day, and carry a well-stocked purse the size of a refrigera-tor. Friends tell me I make it look easy, but I'm still no Fred Astaire.

I Crave, Therefore I Am

by Claire Collins

Before I was diagnosed with diabetes seven years ago, one of my favorite pastimes was baking chocolate chip cookies. After a bad day at work, if I was depressed, lonely, or bored (which is to say, at least once a week), I'd buy a bag of chips and start cooking. By the time the cookies were baked, though, I was so full of the batter that I rarely ate any and would give them away instead.

All that changed overnight, of course, when my doctor told me my sudden weight loss, extreme thirst, and unrelenting fatigue were due to insulin-dependent diabetes.

"Don't worry," he said, probably sensing my distress (I was already kissing my cookies good-bye), "the diet isn't so bad. Just lay off the sweets." It wasn't the last time a doctor tried to minimize what is actually a pretty major lifestyle change.

Had he been honest, he would have told me: "Don't worry. All you have to do is test four times a day, measure and weigh everything you eat, eat at the same time daily, exercise, learn to treat insulin reactions, and take your shots." Had he been honest, I might have gone into a kind of shock that has nothing to do with insulin. While his words served to minimize my plight, they helped me to ease into accepting it.

Actually, I have never minded the testing, or the taking of insulin that this disease requires. For me, a lifelong lover of sweets, all of that has been a piece of, well, cake, com-

pared to sidestepping the cake itself. It's taken a while, but
I've finally come to admit that those cravings aren't likely
to subside completely, just as I still long to own a red
Mercedes sport coupe instead of the station wagon I need
for the family.

There seems, however, to be an assumption, among
doctors, friends, my husband, and my mother, that the
diagnosis of diabetes puts an abrupt halt to any desire for
sweets—or heaping portions of pasta, for that matter.

I am here to tell you that, in my case at least, that
couldn't be further from the truth. I don't think I've passed
a day without fending off a chocolate craving, or the mag-
netic pull of ice cream, or the siren's call of the cookie jar.
Food cravings, it seems, are my lot in life. Whoever said
going weeks without sweets puts an end to sugar lust?

For several years, I dealt with this problem, mostly by
sulking. "You don't want any of this, do you, Claire?"
someone would ask, while cutting into a fudge cheesecake
pie. Don't want any? Don't want any? Not only do I want
some, I want the whole pie, and whipped cream, too. The
fact is, though, I can't have it and no, I'm not going to be a
sport about it. I'm going to leave the room and indulge in a
little moping, thank you.

While I used to regard anyone who ate dessert in front
of me as a traitor, an enemy, a sadist, I can now watch others indulge without wanting to harm them. After seven
years. I have finally accepted my lot. At times, I'm even
able to see the up side, to understand that the way I eat
now is better for me and for my kids, who actually believe
that applesauce is a treat.

Still, it's just so darned hard sometimes to say no. To
ward off cravings, I find myself using tactics that are the

psychological equivalent of wearing a garlic necklace and carrying a cross to repel vampires. I have taped the number 285 to my refrigerator, so that I must stare at it every time I go to get a snack. That's the number my blood sugar rose to the last time I gave in to a chocolate craving.

Often, I'll rifle through my stack of *Diabetes Forecast* magazines, looking for articles about retinopathy or neuropathy or nephropathy, which tend to jolt me into compliance. Sometimes, only emergency measures will do. When I turn off the TV and pull out the stroller, my kids don't even have to ask: They know we're all going out for a walk, fast.

I am only human and sometimes, the cravings are stronger than I am. I have to remind myself that controlling my diabetes is like being in my own 12-step program. I take it one day at a time; I don't let a single slip send me spinning out of dietary control.

Lately, I've even begun to realize that my life really isn't so drastically different from most people's, after all. We've all got a battle to fight, and nobody wins by eating the whole cheesecake. Understanding this helps me feel less singled out, less different from everyone else. My weakness for sweets is part of what makes me human.

Or, to paraphrase the words of a famous philosopher: I crave, therefore I am.

Editor's note: The new dietary guidelines recommend that you have a meal plan developed to fit your lifestyle. Sugar is a carbohydrate that can be included as part of your meal plan.

Finding a Deeper Strength

by John G. Bentley

Fifteen years ago, I was a thirty-something single male living obliviously on the "bachelor diet." This was basically potato chips and anything that could be squirted on them, scooped up by them, or stuck to the little crumbs in the bottom of the bag. I was in hog heaven, sailing serenely down life's lazy river. The last time I'd seen a doctor was at the Army induction physical. Health concerns didn't even form a blip on my horizon.

I'd developed a bit of a gut, so I was delighted when I started losing weight. I had some vague notions that it might have something to do with my insatiable thirst and the midnight trips to the bathroom, and then to the kitchen to chug a quart of milk or soda. Then I started having a daily battle on the drive home to stay awake. I blamed this on my nocturnal treks from bathroom to kitchen. At no point did any of this ring any alarm bells or prompt thoughts of sickness. I felt fine, after all. How could I be sick?

Then my feet started to hurt, and I began to limp. Only when other people started asking what was wrong did it even occur to me that anything *was* wrong. I finally visited a podiatrist, and he tried a variety of things to ease the pain. Finally, he sent me for a blood test. Bingo! My blood glucose was 350 mg/dl. I had type I diabetes.

The news was a kick in the pants. Health was something I just had—it was a given, like fresh air and sunrises.

I was hurt, angry, and ashamed. I didn't feel sick, and yet here I was in my PJs wandering around a hospital (much to the nurses' indignation). I learned how to give an orange a painless shot of water, and then discovered I could give myself a shot of insulin, however unorangelike my love handles were. But I didn't see any point to all this. I just felt used, abused, and totally confused.

OK, my feet did stop hurting, and the afternoon grogginess cleared up, so maybe the daily shots were doing some good. But forever? Come on! I read all the books, I dutifully watched the videos in the doctor's office, but it was taking awhile to sink in. A few bad reactions finally focused my mind: Yes, dude, you have diabetes. Deal with it.

I quickly discovered that bad habits die hard. I tried to go cold turkey on junk food and found that I wasn't the bastion of self-control I thought I was. My capacity for change was lamentably small, so I just made many small changes. I struggled for 3 years to drop one greasy favorite at a time, replacing each with a fresh fruit or veggie. Each change took awhile to stick, but each small victory made the next one that much easier. In the same way, I started to walk for exercise, and slowly built up to a brisk 3-mile walk daily. Gradually, my reactions faded as I and my diet became healthier.

I realized that taking care of myself wasn't self-indulgence—it was self-respect. I had to maintain my body with the same dedication I had in maintaining my car. Ignoring my health was as stupid as driving down the freeway with an engine squeak getting louder and louder: Pull over, fool! I learned to listen to body knocks and psychic pings, and to notice the effect stress had on my blood sugar. I learned to downshift on the curves and drive defensively.

I'd even park now and then and amble out to enjoy the view. Slower is often better. I discovered peace and grew to relish it.

Older isn't always wiser, but as far as my health is concerned, I am wiser now. The "bachelor diet" is long gone, and good riddance. I exercise daily and watch my diet and weight. I don't obsess about my health, but simply stay aware of it as something that deserves watching and

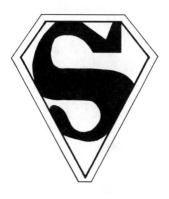

working on.

Diabetes has forced me to become realistic about the world and my place in it. I know now that I'm not invulnerable, and never was (childhood dreams of being Superman to the contrary). I guess it's one of life's little ironies that illness can often make us stronger, at least inside where it counts. Physical strength and good health are important, but transient. Inner strength and good humor last a lifetime.

Luck Isn't Enough

by Rick Fusillo

I am 43 years old and have had insulin-dependent (type I) diabetes for 37 years. I remember my mother crying when the doctor told her that I had diabetes. It was scary for me, seeing my mother react that way. But my family was reassured that with proper precautions, life could be "relatively" normal.

I am living proof of that 1952 statement. Relative, however, is the key word here. As is the case with most people with diabetes, I certainly have had my slumps. A combination of care and luck contributed to the success that I have achieved. I measure my success by the excellent physical and mental condition I am lucky enough to possess currently.

Luck is something you cannot control. Some of us have it, and others don't. Care, however, is something you can control.

As a youngster, I had a lot of luck. I don't remember ever having an insulin reaction, and my blood sugars were always excellent, according to my doctor. When I reflect back on those early years, I realize how much I "lucked out." Every day after school all my buddies went to the local candy store, and of course, I didn't want to be different, so I tagged along. When I remember the "no-no's" I consumed—cherry colas, pound cake, candy bars—it raises my blood sugar just thinking about it.

I was also extremely active. I participated in strenuous sports and activities every day after school and on weekends. I certainly didn't realize it then, but if I hadn't eaten all the "forbidden fruit," I probably would have had many insulin reactions.

Don't get me wrong. This luck does not make it okay. Those were the early, and very lucky, years.

As I moved into my late teens and early 20s, I became a little smarter about how insulin works and how adjustments are made in the dosage. Those were undoubtedly my danger years. I remember taking 65 units of NPH U-80, and waking up in the emergency room on a regular basis.

I went into insulin shock more times than I care to remember, twice in my car. One time I had a head-on collision with a vehicle driven by a woman six months pregnant. Although both cars were totaled, we all escaped serious injury, including the unborn child. Those last three months of her pregnancy were real scary for me, and you can be sure my auto insurance company was as pleased as I when the woman gave birth to a normal, healthy baby.

Another time, I drove past my exit, eventually exited, parked, and passed out. The police found me with no license, no registration, and no identification. (A medical identification tag would have come in real handy.) Because of my unusual behavior, they admitted me to the drug rehabilitation section of a local hospital. In a brief moment of coherence, I told the doctors that I had diabetes. They immediately ran a blood test—my blood sugar had plummeted to 7 mg/dl. The doctor told me this condition could have caused brain damage or even death. When would I learn how important it was to take better care of myself?

As I pressed on into my late 20s and early 30s, I began to take control. What motivated me to change? I was frustrated by my lack of control, especially those all-too-frequent trips to the emergency room. Also, as I grew older, I better appreciated my mortality and wanted to do everything I could to postpone proof of it. Finally, I just wanted the upper hand and decided I would reverse the roles that diabetes and I had taken on—I was now going to control it, rather than have it control me.

It was time to stop relying on luck. It was time to rely on care. Care is something everyone can have, and if you want to increase your chances of a long and healthy life, I believe that care is where the focus should be placed.

I've learned to eat healthier and adjust insulin dosages based on logic, not emotion. I've learned how important exercise is. I even do about five blood tests a day. I feel good about myself. I know I'm in good shape and I like that feeling. After 37 years of type I diabetes, I've been lucky enough to have no complications, nor do I have any signs of any. I see my doctor quarterly, my eye doctor twice a year. I believe it's taken me too many years to "get smart," but, again, I've been one of the lucky ones.

I don't mean to sound as if everything is perfect now, because it's not. It never is with diabetes. Sometimes I feel as if I'm walking a tightrope—not a lot of room for error. I just wish all people with diabetes could have my luck, but I know better. When all is said and done, your odds are much better with care than they are with luck.

I Saw My Future

by Karen Schulz

A good friend of mine called one night in need of advice. She said she'd been feeling bad about herself lately, even taking anti-depressant pills, but she still felt like she couldn't go on. "You've been depressed before," she said to me, "How did you pull out of it?"

I paused. She was referring to my late teen years. Back then, I took all the frustration and anxiety of young adulthood, of my parents' separation, and of maintaining a straight-A average in school out on my health. With all that was going on, I had no time to take care of my diabetes.

How did I do it then, when my blood sugars were consistently higher than my meter could measure and my energy level barely enough to get me off the couch to the bathroom every hour? What got me through the times when, at 19, I felt that I had nothing to live for, that I didn't deserve good health, that I wasn't worth the effort of trying, that I may as well give up?

She was right. I once did fall into a pit of anger, fear, guilt, and depression, and I had to get myself out.

"I guess I saw my future," I told her. "And it wasn't that great."

"What do you mean?" she asked.

"I knew where my behavior was leading me. And I knew I could change it. So I pictured myself, years into the future, how I wanted to be. Everything. What I would look like, what I'd be doing, who I'd be with. I created my ideal self. And then I had something to look forward to."

The silence grew long as she was thinking. "If that fails," I said, "I usually go shopping."

"You're right," she said, laughing. "Look how well you've done. You did have something to look forward to. And it all began with setting your mind to do it."

We hung up, and I just sat for a long time. I couldn't remember a day since I was 7 years old when I didn't think about my diabetes, what I was up against, and what my future held.

I have had to "pull myself out" many times, with every unintentional ice cream binge, every higher-than-we-like-it A_{1c} result, every new complication and drop in self-esteem. I might have deserved an A for effort, but I'd still feel like I'd flunked.

I remember the question, "What motivates you?" coming up in a diabetes support group session that I attended. What surprised me most that night wasn't that everyone gave the same answer, but that every woman in the room said she was motivated by one thing: fear. Fear of blindness, fear of death, fear of mystery and of uncertainty, and of their own bodies.

I realized then how important is the motivation that gets us to take care of diabetes. Most people, at some point in their lives, will claim they're dieting or getting in shape, but usually the goal is short-term, like a high school reunion or a desirable number on the scale.

But diabetes is a daily disease—blood tests, shots, walks, meals of specific size at specific times—on an infinite time line. Years, decades, forever. It takes something very powerful to keep you motivated for that.

I generally don't perform well under negative reinforcement. The night those seven women admitted that fear was what motivated them, I kept trying to picture myself running for my life, trying to escape from the perils of diabetes. But I knew I wouldn't keep up my daily routine that way, with the Cloud of Doom hanging over my head. I had better things to do.

I chose, instead, to picture my future, imagining myself as attractive, healthy, happy, and successful. Then I could run *to* something, rather than *from* something. The world didn't look so frightful. And I could focus my energies in positive ways. I believed in myself.

Eventually, my parents sorted out their problems and went on, and I graduated from college with an A-average. I've also met a doctor who gives me positive encouragement and exceptional attention in controlling my diabetes. (Not that I have perfect control, of course, but my doctor and I have become weekly comrades in an effort to make the highs less high and the lows less frequent.)

Now, every so often, when I find myself drifting from my normally strict regimen and wishing I could crawl into a hole and hide from my diabetes, I think about my friend and that phone call. Then I look at how my future is turning out—what I look like, what I'm doing, and who I'm with. I am strengthened to see how far I have come. And I have high hopes for the future.

Always Thinking

by Dale Frost Stillman

I've always loved school. (Of course, my kids think I'm crazy.) Literature and creative writing were my best subjects. Actually, it's no surprise to me that I'm creative. I have diabetes.

Being creative means approaching a problem with an open mind, observing it from every angle, and then making a decision. Controlling my diabetes also requires such flexibility and thought. Sometimes, I wonder, which came first, the creativity or the diabetes?

I'm not sure I remember. But I do know that having diabetes is a constant exercise in creative thinking and decision making. It is a thinking person's disease. There's no vacation from its challenges, and there are decisions to be made at every turn. My mind must always be alert.

Consider my morning routine. I wake up early, brush my teeth, stick my finger for a blood test, and then inject my morning insulin. That all happens before I've even had my first cup of coffee. (Sound familiar?)

I may have to adjust my dosage of insulin because of my blood test result. Or maybe it's because I'm going jogging that morning, or because I'm late for a meeting and it's breakfast on the run. Whatever the case, I make my calculations and make a decision.

Self-management decisions are not the only challenges diabetes presents to me. There are other problems that are more complex, and take lots of time and thought to resolve.

I have chosen not to hide my diabetes. But making the decision to be so open about this disease was not easy. In fact, it took years to think this through. As a child, while friends contemplated whether to kiss on the first date, I decided whether to discuss diabetes on the first date. In the days prior to disposable syringes, maneuvering a sleepover was a nightmare. My good friends "knew," but who else was I supposed to tell? While others gossiped about Pamela's goofy haircut, I snuck off to the refrigerator, retrieved my pre-drawn syringe, and smuggled it to the bathroom, replete with alcohol wipe and urine testing equipment.

Nowadays, I inject at restaurant tables and freely reveal my diabetes to anyone who cares to listen.

I like to think that the decisions I was forced to make as a child fostered strength of character, which gradually grew into an independent spirit and a strong sense of responsibility. But even with all the wisdom I've gained from living with diabetes, some questions seem impossible to answer. My most pressing question these days is, how do I present diabetes to my children?

A few weeks ago my 12-year-old son, Ryan, had to do a report on a "disabled person." You should have seen the look on his face when he found Mary Tyler Moore's name on the list of potential subjects. "Mommy," he snickered, "she's got diabetes, like you. She's not disabled." I was inclined to pat myself on the back for having had the good sense to downplay diabetes as an illness. But my pride was short-lived when I realized that Ryan obviously did not see the whole picture.

He sees diabetes as normal because I manage my diabetes well and live a normal life. But he hasn't yet realized the effort it takes for me to live this way. He doesn't know that diabetes sometimes causes serious complications. I work this over in my mind and consider the best ways to answer the questions he's bound to ask, once he starts to learn about the uglier side of this disease.

Last week I was checking my blood sugar after dinner, and my youngest son, Travis, happened to be nearby. Travis is a profound thinker (although some of his teachers might be surprised to hear him described that way). "Mommy, will I get diabetes?" he asked as casually as he had asked for another helping of french fries at dinner. "I don't think so, T." Satisfied, he sauntered off after a bowl of ice cream. But I was left thinking again; second guessing the answer I had given him.

These questions are the toughest test of my creative abilities. It seems I'm never quite satisfied with the answers I come up with. Perhaps this is because the best answer I can give my children has less to do with what I say to them than with how I live my life. The best answer I can give my children is to manage my diabetes well and to continue living a healthy life. I'd rather they leave the thinking to me.

Descartes said "I think, therefore I am." I say, "I have diabetes, therefore I think."

Disaster or Challenge?

by Eugenia Fore

My husband loves ice cream. He also loves to serve it to guests. So, on a recent occasion when our son, his wife, and children had dinner with us, everyone waited expectantly to see which exotic flavor Grandpa would serve. Generous portions of chocolate-almond-marshmallow were doled out.

Suddenly our youngest granddaughter, newly turned 2, noticed I had no ice cream in front of me. She turned to her grandfather and exclaimed, "Papa! Papa!"

"Yes, honey?" he asked her.

When she pointed to me and said, "Mama! Mama!" everyone at the table realized that the tender-hearted little girl thought Grandma had been left out.

I was touched and amused at her reaction, because though I think nothing of it now when people eat something I can't have, I recall a time when such occasions left me feeling painfully left out and excluded.

In 1961 I was diagnosed with type I (insulin-dependent) diabetes, known at the time as juvenile diabetes. How could a 34-year-old woman suddenly acquire a juvenile disease?

I had always considered myself safe from diabetes since we knew of no one with diabetes in the family. So I reacted to the diagnosis with shock and dismay. Never having had a weight problem, I couldn't imagine being unable to eat whatever I wanted.

After 10 days in the hospital, I went home, a little scared, but buoyed by the support of my husband and two young children. I was taking 80 units of insulin a day, but with strict adherence to my prescribed regimen, I was soon able to decrease the amount.

As time went by, however, I observed other people with diabetes treating their condition casually, even negligently. I, too, became somewhat careless about food, especially at social gatherings. I did continue to give myself insulin injections faithfully and test my urine fairly regularly. Every six weeks I had a fasting blood sugar test at the doctor's office.

Years passed and I never missed taking my shot, but urine and blood-glucose testing became less and less frequent. My attitude had gradually become one of merely getting by. After all, the tests always came out too high anyway. Why waste time and effort on it? Even with that attitude, I remained under the illusion that I had accepted my condition—until one summer evening in 1976.

The occasion was a church meeting at a friend's home. Entering the kitchen, I noticed a plate of fresh, homemade, chocolate chip cookies. Visions of their chewy, chocolatey goodness captivated me all evening, so it was quite a letdown when the hostess presented me not with a cookie, but with a large, Golden Delicious apple.

Knowing my friend meant well, I accepted it with mumbled thanks, but anger seethed within me. "How dare she assume I can't have a cookie like everyone else? Don't I have as much right as they do?" Later, I sneaked a couple of cookies.

The taste lived up to my expectations but eating them did not bring the anticipated pleasure. Instead, I was displeased with what I suddenly knew to be a foolish, futile attitude.

I lay awake long into the night, shocked by the vehemence of my anger. Realizing that I'd never accepted the condition I'd been living with for 15 years and that I actually resented people who didn't have diabetes, I asked God to forgive me and help me make a fresh start.

I resolved to accept that I had diabetes and to view it not as a disaster, but as a challenge. Changing old habits took time, but each small success paved the way for the next.

I was soon rewarded, not only with improved health, but with a deep sense of accomplishment. My biggest surprise came when I let go of my unrealistic dreams of "off-limit" foods, and I began to eat fruits and vegetables. I found out I like them!

I am now on a strict diet—low levels of sodium, fat, and cholesterol. But because I had learned to live with restrictions, I eased into these with very little difficulty.

I marvel at the advances in knowledge and technology that make it possible for people with diabetes to monitor their blood glucose by themselves several times a day.

And when my monitoring tells me it's time for a midafternoon snack, guess what I eat and enjoy? You got it—a cool, crisp, crunchy apple!

Editor's note: The new dietary guidelines recommend that you have a meal plan developed to fit your lifestyle. Sugar is a carbohydrate that can be included as part of your meal plan.

Letting Go of the Labels

by Ruth T. Stingley

W hen I was in the second grade, I had to wear a sign on my back that read: "I HAVE BAD MANNERS." In an attempt to teach our class proper etiquette, our misguided teacher handed out a list of all the rules we had to follow to demonstrate good manners. If we violated any of these rules, we had to wear the dreaded sign. I twice neglected to thank my teacher for giving me papers to hand out; and for one whole week, I bore "I HAVE BAD MANNERS" on my back.

As a teacher myself some 20 years later, I know that positive comments motivate children more strongly than pinning embarrassing signs on their backs. Too many children—and adults—have labels burned into their subconscious.

People with diabetes are no exception. I know. I am finally trying to cast off the heavy labels I carry with me because I have diabetes.

When I was diagnosed with diabetes at the age of 14, I wasn't exactly thrilled, but I attempted to learn all I could about the disease. My two daily shots were not nearly as difficult as the urine testing proved to be. Before every meal and bedtime, I "voided," then drank as many glasses of water as I could stomach. After half an hour, I "voided" again, catching some urine into my trusty blue container.

Then came the real test of discipline. So many drops of urine, so many drops of water, and the plop of the test tablet. And, for one long, demanding year—for 1,408 tests—the fizzing mixture turned bright orange. Although I followed my diet, took my tests, injected my insulin, and called my doctor every morning, my urine turned that hated orange, which meant that it contained a high amount of sugar. Throughout the course of that year, a "FAILURE" sign slowly strung itself around my neck.

After a year of complete compliance and diligence, and only negative test results, I ditched the testing. Now I realize that it's only human nature to give up in the face of such odds. Try any person on this earth: Make him follow strict guidelines that separate him from his peers, then test and flunk him four times a day, every day for a year. At the time, though, I didn't understand that I was reacting in a normal way. I was a "failure."

I fabricated test results in my log book for the doctor, which made me a liar. I occasionally wavered on my diet, which made me a cheat. In my mind, all the world could plainly see the horrendous labels prominently displayed on my back: FAILURE, LIAR, CHEAT.

At age 18, I resolved to make amends for my "criminal behavior," and I followed a low-calorie diet and an exercise plan. Yet my urine tests still turned orange. My doctor called me a "liar" to my face. "You are cheating on your diet," he proclaimed from behind a small podium in his office. I never went back to him; the damage was done.

I denied my disease and strove for perfection in other areas of my life. Yet I could never be good enough at anything, for deep inside, I carried those awful labels with me.

At age 26, I used a blood glucose meter for the first time and learned that I could have some semblance of control over my diabetes. Once again I became diligent, and this time I began to see favorable results. But the labels were still there.

Three years later, I found myself fighting another label. It was slapped on me when my daughter was born with a birth anomaly. I knew my diabetes was not responsible, for I had been in excellent control throughout the entire pregnancy, but the reactions of others made me feel once again like that 14-year-old girl who couldn't seem to get anything right.

Out on my morning walk one day, I stopped in my tracks, tears flowing beneath my sunglasses. I didn't care what the passersby thought. I was crying for that little girl in me who was overwhelmed by those signs. "You're okay," I told the child inside me. "You're not a failure, not a liar, not a cheat."

And suddenly, I realized that it wasn't just me. Scores of people with diabetes, children and adults alike, have been slapped with negative labels that only compound the problem. We need to be told that we have courage and strength of character. We face an illness every day that can't always be controlled by following strict guidelines, one that allows no vacations and grants no respite.

We need to let go of those horrendous labels and proudly proclaim, "We are 'SURVIVORS.' "

Friends and Lovers

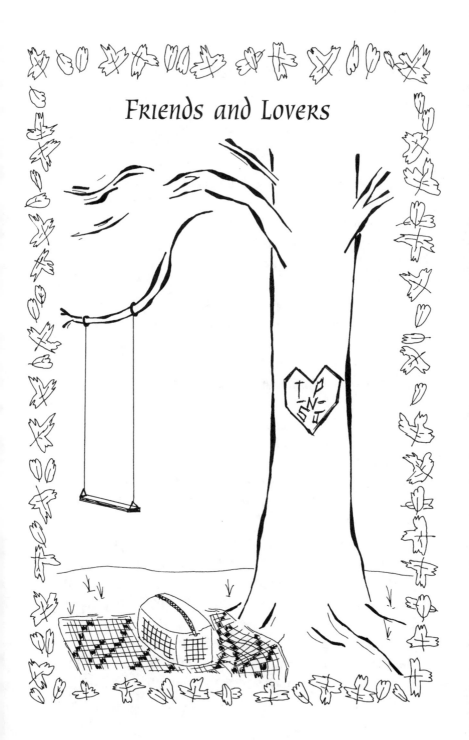

Dog Therapy

by Lisa L. Swope

Whenever my sisters and I asked for a dog, my parents recited the list of reasons we shouldn't get one, and we responded why we should.

Them: It would get hit by a car.

Us: But we could keep it inside.

Them: Dogs shed.

Us: We will vacuum. Every day.

Them: Who will feed the dog and take care of it when it is sick?

Us: We will. We'll take turns.

It never worked. Our parents' reasons were well-grounded in reality, and we knew, as they knew, that vacuuming and cleaning up accidents on the rug were jobs children wouldn't do for very long.

Then it happened. I was lying in a hospital bed, when my parents leaned over and whispered, "Just name anything in the world you want, sweetheart, and when you get out of the hospital, we'll get it for you."

Sure, getting diabetes and spending 13 days of my summer vacation in the hospital when I was only 11 had been a rotten break, but my parents' concerned faces looking down at me promising anything I wanted was a fantasy come true.

"I want a dog," I said. My parents' faces sank, but their eyes held their promise. It might take a few months of negotiations, but in my heart, I knew I had my dog.

Their terms were few: It couldn't shed; and if it cost money, my sisters and I would have to pay for it. That was the week my sister's friend, Mary Bane, got a poodle puppy. Her parents were very strict; they had a no shedding rule, too.

"There are two puppies left," Mom told us when she got off the phone, "but they cost $50. If you can find the money, I guess you can have one."

We climbed the stairs to our bedroom and sat on the floor. "How can we come up with $50?" I asked.

"We could save our allowances," my youngest sister Leslie suggested.

"By the time we had enough money, the dog would be gone," Freddi said.

We emptied our pockets, and the loose change between us came to less than a dollar.

"We could use the Kennedy-head bank," Freddi said.

On our shelf sat a huge plastic bank in the shape of a Kennedy-head half dollar. "Mom," we said, "could we have a knife to open our bank?"

"Ralph," she said to our father, "I think the girls are getting a dog."

What a dog! Except for his white face, paws, and "bow tie" patch on his neck, Renni was black. His hair (not fur—he didn't shed) was curly and soft. He followed my bike, licked my tears, and waited patiently by the windowsill for me to come home. He was the only friend I had who understood how I felt about my diabetes.

My diabetes wouldn't stay at home. It followed me to school, to pajama parties, and to the pool. My friends asked why I sometimes had to stop swimming suddenly and have a snack, or why I had to change my lunch or why I couldn't have a sip of their colas. Every kid wants to be unique, but nobody wants to be different. I was different.

Renni's friendship, however, was unconditional. He never stared at me when I took my shot; he never asked questions about my diet or insulin reactions. When it was easy to sit in my room and feel sorry for myself, Renni's paw scratched at my bedroom door and summoned me outside. His tail wagged as I laced up my sneakers, and he followed me faithfully on my bike through the neighborhood.

The night after I left for college, Renni looked for me. He roamed the hills near our house and returned the next morning tired and dirty. Most weekends I went home and on those mornings I woke to his tail wagging.

I was 28 and a high school teacher when my parents had to put Renni to sleep. He was a few months shy of 17. "Old enough to drive," I would tell my high school students, "nearly old enough to buy beer and vote." My blood sugars soared that week.

Dogs can't cure diabetes. But Renni helped me focus on something other than myself and he helped me come to terms with my diabetes.

Once, when my mother was reminiscing about Renni, she said, "You know, we got him in 1970. Most of the loose change you bought him with was real silver. Can you imagine how much it would be worth now?" But things like that are relative, I guess. Renni and me, we shared our youth together. And Renni—chasing butterflies, licking my tears, running alongside my bike with an early evening summer breeze in our faces—was worth his weight in gold to me.

Twenty Years and Counting

by Barbara Ryan, RD, MPH

My favorite T-shirt is old, worn, and unraveling around the edges. It's comfortably shabby now and it's been on my mind a lot. Powdermilk Biscuits is emblazoned on the front. Anyone familiar with the radio show "Prairie Home Companion" and the mythical town of Lake Wobegone, knows about powdermilk biscuits. They are a most important part of life there, because they "give you the strength to do what needs to be done."

I have lived 20 years with insulin-dependent diabetes and what has had to be done is four shots of insulin and two blood tests a day. It requires vigilance 24 hours a day. Although I have, at times, felt triumphant—ready to "leap tall buildings with a single bound," other times I've felt like I was carrying a huge burden uphill. I have needed those powdermilk biscuits.

I was introduced to injections and diet by a physician who believed that if you don't make a big deal out of it, then it won't be a big deal. He sat me down in his office and told me that I'd have to take a shot every day. He filled the syringe, pointed to my leg, and said, "Just a quick jab. That's all there is to it." And I believed him.

Then he tore off a diet from a pad, handed it to me, and told me to follow it. That was it. No big deal.

I went home. My mother cried when she heard the news, but my tears came gradually, with each insulin reaction, each time I felt lousy, each time I felt what "no big deal" was.

In six months, I was off to college and my control "roller coastered." My weight skyrocketed on the 2,200-calorie diet the doctor gave me. I was a regular at the emergency room. And most alarmingly, I discovered the negative attitudes some people harbor about diabetes.

In the third year following my diagnosis, I chose to write a paper for a nutrition class. I wanted to find out how students with diabetes were managing with the food served in the dining halls. Much to my surprise, I couldn't locate anyone with diabetes on campus. Because of confidentiality concerns, health services wouldn't release any names to me. So I worked by word of mouth.

One woman I contacted hurried me to her room, closed the door, and made it very clear she wanted no one to know of her diabetes. It would, she was sure, affect friendships and her whole future. I didn't understand her attitude. I didn't believe that diabetes was like leprosy, so my friends didn't treat me like it was. Looking back, I realize that my family and friends have been my powder-milk biscuits from the beginning.

When I began injecting myself with insulin, I used a glass syringe with disposable needles. I tested my urine for sugar with tape and for ketones with a fizzing tablet. I took one shot of insulin a day that tied me to rigid mealtimes. The few articles I could find to read on diabetes were dull and somber.

Each new year, however, has brought new developments that have profoundly affected my life. Disposable syringes, improved quality insulins, normalization of the diabetic diet, and glucose self-monitoring (the best biscuit since sliced bread), have all lightened my burden.

But even though diabetes has been gentle with me, I still feel as tattered as my T-shirt. Although I have the advantage of being a dietitian and having access to good medical care, my knowledge doesn't always translate into good choices. Knowing the exchange system inside out just causes a huge guilt trip when I don't do the right thing. Knowing isn't doing, and it's the doing that makes me tired.

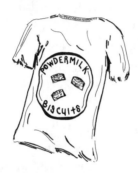

So at this 20-year mark I have been forced to admit to myself and others how weary I am of diabetes. Every time I do, I feel better. It's like I've gotten a biscuit every time someone else understands, on some level, what it means to have diabetes.

To my great surprise, my honest expression of need has resulted in a generous showing of support. Two friends treated me to a 20-year celebration, with dinner, poems, special gifts, and a trip to the theater to show their friendship and solidarity with me. In this loving celebration, they created a ritual of real sharing.

Funny, my burden is still there. I know all that I have to do. But I think I have found a fresh supply of those powdermilk biscuits.

One is a Lonely Number

by Bonnie Wheeler

It was my first week on a new job, and I was waiting for a meeting to start. "One sure is a lonely number," I thought to myself. Then the friendly nurse sitting next to me introduced herself, "Hi, I'm Trish! What's your Medic Alert bracelet for?" (I assume questions like this must come more easily in a medical group.) We discovered that not only were we both new employees, but we shared type II diabetes and taking insulin, too.

When my diabetes was first diagnosed, my doctor gave me basic instructions and turned me loose. The label "diabetes" and the thought of daily injections were scary enough, but the absolute aloneness I felt was terrifying. It was 10 years after my diagnosis before I met another person with diabetes.

Over the next year, Trish and I became a support group of two. "Hey, Bonnie, I had a hypoglycemic reaction last night. Have you ever had your lips go numb?" "Trish, at night my feet feel like they're on fire, and I can hardly get to sleep, have you ever...?"

Trish and I know about diabetes: She has taught patients about diabetes in her more than 20 years of nursing, and I researched diabetes with the same thoroughness that I would a professional writing assignment. So, if she and I felt the need for mutual support, what about all the diabetic patients who come to our medical group? How do they handle "Have you ever...?"

With that question in mind, I approached our administrator with a formal proposal for the medical group to sponsor a diabetes support group. Shortly after my proposal was approved, *Diabetes Forecast* ran an article (June 1991, pp. 54–60) on "Starting a Support Group." Using the article as my guide, I contacted our local ADA affiliate, called existing groups in my area, started building a resource file, and developed a schedule. We planned a mix of activities involving outside speakers and mutual support meetings.

From the beginning, refreshments were an important part of the program. One of the most common complaints (especially with newly diagnosed people) is: "I feel so deprived—I can never have dessert again!" A member who was having a bout with steroid-induced diabetes was also a gourmet baker. She used her expertise to develop special "legal" desserts for our group; no one ever feels "deprived" at our meetings. Monthly refreshments, a potluck dinner, and a picnic have shown us that good food and social events can be compatible with diabetes.

Support groups are about people. When the group started, I thought, "What can I do to help these people?" But as the group took on a life of its own, I found that I was being taught and supported as well.

Half of our 30 members are patients at our medical group and half come from the local community. Our ages vary from 25 to 80. We have members with type I and members with type II, those who are newly diagnosed and those who have had diabetes for 35 years. Our common ground is our diagnosis, our desire to learn, and our concern for one another.

Our gourmet baker moved, so other members volunteer to bring refreshments. Elynor makes reminder calls to everyone each month. None of us allows other members to sit in a corner alone; one of us always goes to them. When I am tempted to go off my program, I think of the group. The group helps keep me on track because there is no such thing as denial when someone is watching. Through contacting the speakers and digging up educational material for the group, I am learning every day.

I continue to be inspired by the sheer guts and determination of the people in our support group. Gary has had numerous severe hypoglycemic reactions and keeps looking for answers. Carol has had diabetes for 30 years, and her husband says, "I am part of this group, because we are looking for answers to our problem." Pat is newly diagnosed and full of fear and questions. Julie (at age 25, the baby of our group) has had diabetes since she was 9 months old and is on a waiting list for pancreas and kidney transplants. One married couple, Ernie and Lynda, both strive to keep their diabetes under control while caring for their large family of foster children.

Our group meeting is the joy of my month. It inspires me, educates me, and shows me that diabetes is a bump in the road of life—not a dead end. One is still a lonely number, but there is strength in numbers.

Editor's note: The new dietary guidelines recommend that you have a meal plan developed to fit your lifestyle. Sugar is a carbohydrate that can be included as part of your meal plan.

Beyond Survival

by Gloria Schramm

My husband, Fred, rushed through the door one night three months ago, not long after a physical examination.

"I've got it," he declared glibly. I thought he was joking. Then he identified himself as "type II, 364 blood sugar count" and held up a bottle of glyburide.

So there he was, 42 years old, obese for most of his life (though I never saw him that way), and now facing a challenge. This challenge could call him to rise and grow into his best self, or it could sap his will to enjoy life.

And there I was, shaking. I extended heartfelt sympathy and pledged unconditional support, promising to go with him to his dietary classes. I am thankful that my weight-conscious friends taught me how to measure food and gave me a scale. I was never a great-shakes gourmet or "culinary calculator." Survival makes people acclimate, fast.

Although Fred seemed to cope well, a black cloud hovered above me. He had always been an evening couch potato enjoying incessant munching and soda-drinking by the TV. He used to describe himself as a Roman Emperor who just loved to eat, period. How could my husband stand a lifetime of no longer enjoying unlimited quantities of food? What a cruel fate. Worst of all, what if the medicine and diet did not work? What if his blood sugars didn't respond?

But I kept quiet and rose to arms. It might as well have been me. I read and then I read some more. I groped to understand the chemistry of what goes awry in the human body and hoped for a wonder drug that would make his pancreas produce more insulin, or that would make his body access the insulin correctly.

After two long weeks, Fred's blood sugar finally dropped down to a whopping low of 96. He steadily lost three pounds of weight a week. Things were definitely looking up.

Then, as if to dispel any doubts I might still have had about Fred's coping, I had a dream. In the dream, there was an obese man lying drowned at the bottom of a ravine. He was wearing a gold wedding band on his left hand. I didn't know the man, but I knew somebody loved him, and I wanted so badly to rescue him. Fred was there too, stand-ing next to me, and he looked down on this man and shook his head in utter disgust. He dissuaded me from rescuing the man, insisting that he was dead and it was too late.

In the same dream, Fred introduced me to some slim guy I didn't know, but I was very attracted to this fellow. Then it occurred to me that this handsome stranger was Fred.

I marvel, as do our friends, relatives, and co-workers, at how well Fred has adjusted to this new lifestyle. He has now lost more than 40 pounds (and still going) and is assembling a new wardrobe. He's content to watch me squeeze every ounce of fat from turkey burgers. He walks over two miles in an hour—outpacing me on the world-renowned Jones Beach Long Island Boardwalk. His doctor has taken him off glyburide and his blood count has remained normal.

I commend Fred for keeping his spirits up and getting the job done. He says, matter-of-factly, that he had his fun and now the party is over. He never takes his eye off the goal: To be off the medication. His will is palpable. It just goes to show you that survival is a motivator.

But we are also grateful to Fred's doctor and dietitian for their support. The dietitian's road map was invaluable in pointing us in the direction of menu planning and food preparation. Fred can't munch much at night anymore so he chomps on sugarless gum. And he does something else: He talks to me now more than before. After 21 years of marriage, it appears we have a love that endures and transcends adverse circumstances. He has always been loving and supportive of me, and now he's showing his love for me, and himself, in a new and exciting way. I'm very grateful. I can't thank Fred enough for his caring enough to take care of himself.

Fred's thirst was quenched at the oasis of new life. We thought the party was over, but in a way, it has just begun, and the host is a slim, svelte, vibrant man. We can't predict the future, but our faith in God will buoy us along.

WHY ME?

by Ramona Goldman

It was awful. I hated being there, lying in a hospital bed at the age of 27. I could hardly recognize myself in the mirror, weighing in at a mere 72 pounds. And I had trouble comprehending the horrifying words I heard coming out of the mouth of my doctor: "You have diabetes, Ramona."

Everything he said after that point might as well have been spoken to the wall. My then husband-to-be, Richard, was sitting next to my bed, my parents alongside. Could they translate the doctor's message for me? What was going on?

Just a short three months before I had weighed 40 pounds more, and was recovering from respiratory problems and injuries from an auto accident. But this was something else again. My hands shook so badly, I couldn't hold onto a cup. I was experiencing incredible thirst and nausea, which my physician at first thought could have been caused by my pain medication. And now this, those doctor's words: "You have diabetes." I thought to myself, *I don't want to live like this. Why me?*

Over the next few days I was taught how to give myself injections and how to test my blood glucose levels. Slowly but surely, my appetite came back, and so did my weight.

But there were little things that had changed about me; things I hated. My vision had become blurry and I couldn't read labels on boxes or drive myself to the store. I was told that it would take some time for these conditions to improve because of my high glucose levels, and I felt angry and impatient. Whenever I was alone, I would cry about my new way of life and the struggle I faced adjusting to the daily routine.

Richard called several times a day, not always knowing what to expect as I swung between bouts of triumph and tears. He bought me a pair of extremely strong dime-store magnifying glasses, so I could see well enough to fill my syringes and read a label. Together, we attended diabetes classes at the hospital and gathered all the information we could to better understand this disease. In time, my glucose levels improved, and in turn, so did my vision. Slowly, the pieces of our lives came back together.

Many months later, as I sat across the table from Richard while he carefully drew the insulin for my dinner injection, I realized I was not alone in my anguish. Across from me sat my nurse, my supporter, my emotional bodyguard, my confidant, my one-man support group. As I watched him doing this task that had become second nature, I felt overwhelmed. Here was the one person who knew my triumphs and my pain.

There had been long days for him, when I had been too ill or too weak to comb my hair or to dress myself. There were times my rage erupted like a volcano as I dealt with hopelessness and despair, knowing I would never be the same person I was before. There were also long nights when my blood sugars would drop rapidly. Richard instinctively woke when he thought my breathing seemed irregular or my body felt clammy. There were nights when he rushed to the refrigerator for juice and helped me hold the glass when I shook so badly I couldn't hold it myself. He took countless trips with me to the doctors and specialists. He encouraged me to take charge and to speak up when I felt a treatment wasn't meeting my needs.

I had become so accustomed to his faithful support that I never realized how difficult it would have been for me if he hadn't been there by my side. I had never once considered the impact my diabetes had on him. On some days, he carried the burden of this illness when I felt I could not. He never hinted that he was unsure of our lives together or that we couldn't handle the obstacles this disease created.

It's now been three years since that day at the dinner table. I no longer think of diabetes as a burden, but as a way of life. And as with anything in our lives, some times are good and others are trying.

I think we all draw strength from somewhere deep inside where we've saved it up until that very moment when we need it most. This strength is grounded in love and faith. These are found in the simplest acts: a few words of support or kindness, or that careful filling of a syringe by someone who wants to assure you that you don't have to go it alone.

As I sit across that same table and look at the man who has given so much, sacrificed so much, and nurtured so much, I once again ask *Why me?* But this time, my grateful heart requires no response.